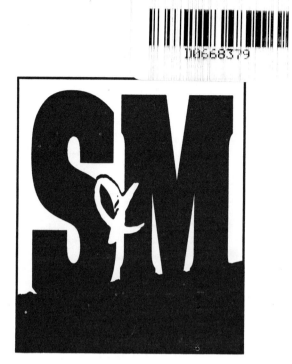

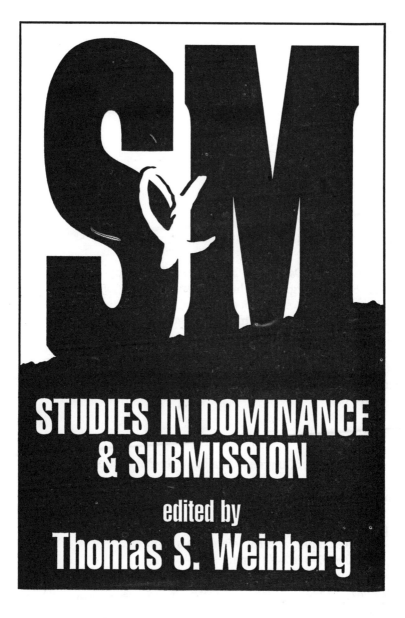

S&M

STUDIES IN DOMINANCE & SUBMISSION

edited by

Thomas S. Weinberg

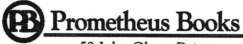

Prometheus Books

59 John Glenn Drive
Amherst, NewYork 14228-2197

Published 1995 by Prometheus Books

99 98 97   5 4 3

Library of Congress Cataloging-in-Publication Data

S and M : studies in dominance and submission. — Rev. ed. / edited
    by Thomas S. Weinberg.
    p.   cm.
    Includes bibliographical references and index.
    ISBN 0-8797-5-978-X (paper)
    1. Sadomasochism. I. Weinberg, Thomas S.
HQ79.S23   1995
306.77'5—dc20   95-12356

                                                          CIP

Printed in the United States of America on acid-free paper

For my wife, Bonnie,
with love

Preface

A dozen years ago, the late G. W. Levi Kamel and I coedited our first volume on sadomasochism. We felt that the most prevalent view of sadomasochists at that time was the psychodynamic position and that the sociological perspective on S&M had not been widely disseminated. We believed that viewing S&M as a subculture, with its own norms, values, and symbols, added importantly to a balanced scientific understanding of sadomasochism. We emphasized in our own work and in our selection of the writings of other researchers, that S&M could best be understood in terms of erotic dominance and submission, framed within the context of fantasy.

Since the publication of the first book, there has been an increase in sociological writing on S&M. Some of the earlier ideas we had, for example, about the lack of participation of nonprostitute women in the scene, were wrong. Other observations, accurate at the time, are no longer valid because like any other subculture, the world of S&M is constantly changing. Thus, there is a need for a new collection of more recent research on sadomasochism.

In this volume I have retained those articles that I believe to be timeless. Some of them have been shifted to new sections as I looked at them again with the benefit of hindsight. I have included seven new papers that expand our knowledge of and theorizing about S&M. This book includes more ethnographic research and the findings from two surveys of S&Mers.

Thomas S. Weinberg
Buffalo, N.Y.

STATEMENTS
CLASSIC PERSPECTIVES ON SADOMASOCHISM

Thomas S. Weinberg
and G. W. Levi Kamel

S&M: An Introduction to the Study of Sadomasochism

What Is Sadomasochism?

"Sadomasochism" (S&M) is a combined term that has tradition-ally been used for the giving and receiving of pain for erotic gratification. As we shall see, however, such a simple definition is inadequate for describing what is really a very complex type of behavior. "Sadism" and "masochism" were first used in some consistent scientific way by the psychoanalyst Richard von Krafft-Ebing. In *Psychopathia Sexualis*, which first appeared in 1885, Krafft-Ebing defined sadism as "the experience of sexual [*sic*] pleasurable sensations (including orgasm) produced by acts of cruelty, bodily punishment afflicted on one's own person or when witnessed by others, be they animals or human beings." He went on to say that "it may also consist of an innate desire to humiliate, hurt, wound, or even destroy others in order thereby to create sexual pleasure in one's self" (Krafft-Ebing 1965, p. 53). Krafft-Ebing pointed out that sadism occurred frequently among the "sexual perversions" but he further noted that lovers

---

Specially written for this volume.

and young married couples often engaged in some sort of "horseplay," teasing, biting, pinching, and, wrestling "just for fun." Thus, even the roots of extreme displays of sadism were to be found in normal sexual activity. "The transition from these atavistic manifestations, which no doubt belong to the sphere of physiological sexuality, to the most monstrous acts of destructions of the consort's life can be readily traced," he maintained (p. 53). The term *sadism* itself is derived from the Marquis de Sade, a French nobleman and writer who lived during the eighteenth and early nineteenth centuries. Many of de Sade's novels and stories, including *Justine* and *Juliette*, equate cruelty, pain, and humiliation with sexual pleasure.

Krafft-Ebing derived the term *masochism* from the name of Leopold von Sacher-Masoch, whose novels, such as *Venus in Furs*, reflected his personal erotic preoccupation with pain, humiliation, and submission. By "masochism," Krafft-Ebing meant,

> a peculiar perversion of the psychical sexual life in which the individual affected, in sexual feeling and thought, is controlled by the idea of being completely and unconditionally subject to the will of a person of the opposite sex; of being treated by this person as by a master, humiliated and abused. This idea is colored by lustful feeling; the masochist lives in fantasies, in which he creates situations of this kind and often attempts to realize them. (p. 86)

Krafft-Ebing's description of masochism is much more detailed and broader than his definition of sadism. He defines masochism not only in terms of the receiving of pain; but also, and most importantly, he recognizes the centrality of fantasy and the nonphysical aspects of dominance and submission to sadomasochistic relationships.

Sigmund Freud, Krafft-Ebing's contemporary, also wrote extensively on sadism and masochism. Like Krafft-Ebing, Freud recognized the existence of sadism in "the normal individual." "The sexuality of most men," he wrote, shows an admixture of aggression, of a desire to subdue, the biological significance of which lies in the necessity for overcoming the resistance of the sexual object by actions other than *mere* courting. Sadism would then correspond to an aggressive component of the sexual instinct which has become independent and exaggerated and has been brought to the foreground by displacement. (Freud 1938, p. 569)

Although Freud and Krafft-Ebing felt that sadism, in its less extreme forms, was understandable in terms of normal male sexuality, they had a much more difficult time in accepting the possible normalcy of masochism, at least among men. Freud considered masochism to be "further removed from the normal sexual goal than its opposite. It may even be doubted whether it ever is primary and whether it does not more often originate through transformation from sadism" (1938, p. 569). Krafft-Ebing was less explicit than Freud, but a careful reading of *Psychopathia Sexualis* leaves the reader with little doubt that he considered passivity to be less natural for men (but perhaps not for women) than sexual aggression. He writes, "by this perversion his [the male's] sexual instinct is often made more or less insensible to the normal charms of the opposite sex—incapable of a normal sexual life—psychically impotent" (Krafft-Ebing 1965, p. 86).

Unlike Krafft-Ebing, Freud saw sadism and masochism as being two forms of the same entity, and he noted that they were often found in the same person:

He who experiences pleasure by causing pain to others in sexual relations is also capable of experiencing pain in sexual relations as pleasure. A sadist is simultaneously a masochist, though either the active or the passive side of the perversion may be more strongly developed in him and thus, represent his preponderant sexual activity. (Freud 1938, p. 570)

Freud's observation is verified by a number of writers whose articles appear in the present collection. Breslow et al. (1985) and Moser and Levitt (1987), for example, note that many people in the S&M world define themselves as "flexible" or "switchable" in role choice, a definition that made it easier for them to adapt to a variety of partners. Pat Califia, an avowed "sadist," nevertheless reports that she occasionally enjoys taking the masochistic role; and G. W. Levi Kamel points out in his article on gay "leathersex" that "the most exciting S has also served as an M, and the best M is capable of the S role. It is common for an S to have once been an M almost exclusively, and most leathermen begin their sexual lives as slaves" (Kamel 1980, p. 183).

Havelock Ellis claimed in *Studies in the Psychology of Sex* that the distinction made between sadism and masochism is artificial. He argued that this division does not correspond with reality and that "sadism and masochism may be regarded as complementary emotional states; they can not be regarded as opposed states" (Ellis 1942, vol. 1, part 2, p. 159).

Ellis narrowed the definition of sadomasochism used by Krafft-Ebing and Freud; he made reference to "pain" rather than "cruelty." Erotically motivated pain was, for Ellis, the essence of sadomasochism. He preferred the term "algolagnia," which refers specifically to the connection between sexual excitement and pain, to "sadism" and "masochism." In an important modification of Freud and Krafft-Ebing, Ellis not only rejected the idea that sadomasochism was based upon cruelty, but, most importantly, he also believed that much of this behavior was actually motivated by love:

> When we understand that it is pain only, and not cruelty, that is the essential in this group of manifestations we begin to come nearer to their explanation. The masochist desires to experience pain, but he generally desires that it should be inflicted in love; the sadist desires to inflict pain, but in some cases, if not in most, he desires that it should be felt as love. (Ellis 1942, vol. 1, part 2, p. 160)

Ellis also noted that "sadists" limit their "love of pain" to sexual situations—an important point that is taken up by some of the writers in the present book—and that the sadist is concerned with the sexual pleasure of the "victim." In fact, he wrote, "the sadist by no means wishes to exclude the victim's pleasure, and may even regard that pleasure as essential to his own satisfaction" (1942, vol. 1, part 2, p. 166). In this work, Ellis foreshadowed later writers who viewed sadomasochistic situations in terms of social interaction; he noted that sadists do take into account the responses of their masochists. Yet, in a number of important respects, Ellis failed to understand the essence of S&M as a *social behavior*. First of all, he saw the masochist as essentially a passive participant in the situation. He even referred to the masochist as a "victim." Actually, however, S&M scenarios are *willingly and cooperatively* produced; more often than not it is the *masochist's* fantasies that are acted out. Many S&Mers claim, therefore, that the masochist, rather than the sadist, is really in control during a sadomasochistic episode. The partners jointly limit their mutual activities and these restrictions are rarely exceeded. Sadists who are known to disregard previously agreed upon limits are avoided and quickly find themselves without partners.

Ellis missed the essence of S&M in another way. Although the concept of cruelty was correctly eliminated from his definition, Ellis's concomitant limitation of sadomasochism to pain indicates that he knew very little about what actually happens during S&M scenes. Much S&M involves very little pain. Rather, many sadomasochists prefer acts such as verbal humiliation or abuse, cross-dressing, being tied up (bondage), mild spankings where no severe discomfort is involved, and the like. Often, it is the notion of being helpless and subject to the will of another that is sexually titillating. It is the illusion of violence, rather than violence itself, that is frequently arousing to both sadists and masochists. At the very core of sadomasochism is not pain but the idea of control—dominance and submission. Krafft-Ebing, of course, knew this. Nevertheless, both he and Freud still considered sadomasochism to be a "perversion." One of the important contributions Ellis made was to avoid using that term when writing about S&M. In this regard, he seems more objective than a number of other psychoanalytically oriented writers. Both Frank Caprio (1955) and Wilhelm Stekel (1965), for example, viewed sadomasochism solely as an individual psychopathology. Their work was confined to the presentation and psychiatric analysis of case histories.

In 1969, anthropologist Paul Gebhard published what was to become a classic article on "Fetishism and Sadomasochism," which represented a real advance in the study of S&M. Gebhard emphasized that this behavior occurs within a cultural context:

> Sadomasochism is embedded in our culture since our culture operates on the basis of dominance-submission relationships, and aggression is socially valued. Even our gender relationships have been formulated in a framework conducive to sadomasochism: the male is supposed to be dominant and aggressive sexually and the female reluctant or submissive. (p. 77)

Gebhard's belief that sexual aggressiveness and passivity were a product of culture rather than biology represented a significant break from the physiologically motivated theories of Krafft-Ebing and Freud. Having rooted sadomasochism firmly in culture, Gebhard went on to discuss it as a social behavior. He noted at least four features of this behavior that are directly relevant to understanding S&M as a social phenomenon. First, he discussed the prevalence of S&M in literate societies. Second, he noted the symbolic nature of S&M. Third, he implicitly couched sadomasochism in terms associated with interaction (i.e., interaction between sadist and masochist) and context (emphasizing the importance of social milieu). Finally, and perhaps most insightfully, Gebhard conceptualized S&M activity as scripted behavior.

Gebhard's work illustrates the complexity of sadomasochism. It is not merely a manifestation of individual mental illness, nor is it definable in a single sentence. S&M is, most of all, subcultural social behavior. The variations and "richness" of this subculture, with its own special set of norms and values, language, justifications, even publications and formally structured organizations, are amply described in many of the selections in this volume. Sadomasochism is a sexual lifestyle, one to which notions of dominance and submission are central. It is characterized by socially produced and shared fantasies. For many devotees, sadomasochism is play; it is recreational.

Why Should We Study Sadomasochism?: S&M as Social Behavior

The importance of devoting serious study to sadomasochism lies in the social nature of this behavior. If, as Paul Gebhard suggested, S&M has its basis in the culture of the larger society, then an examination of this behavior should help us to better understand certain selected aspects of that culture. In a subculture involving S&M, where behavior often takes "extreme" forms, the cultural assumptions underlying human action should be more visible and explicit than is the case in the larger society. In the sadomasochistic world many of the conventional niceties, which normally obscure motives and interests, are stripped away. Hence, the microcosm of interrelationships and social meanings surrounding, for example, dominance and submission, aggression and passivity, and masculinity and femininity should be more amenable to study than they usually are within the larger culture. It is probably not inaccurate to say that hat we assume to be "normal" configurations of these qualities are neither normal, inevitable, nor immutable. We find, for example, that in the world of the sadomasochist, there is nothing "abnormal" about a male being passive and submissive. He is not necessarily defined by other S&Mers, nor does he have to define himself as unmasculine because he happens to prefer the "bottom" role. A number of writers in the present book note that this is true (e.g., Weinberg 1978; Kamel 1980) and attempt theoretically to account for it.

Studying S&M as a social behavior enables us to probe the nature of a number of other phenomena. Gebhard pointed out that fantasy is extremely important to sadomasochistic encounters. "The average sadomasochistic session is usually scripted," he wrote, "the masochist must allegedly have done something meriting punishment, there must be threats and suspense before the punishment is meted out, etc. Often the phenomenon reminds one of a planned ritual or theatrical production" (Gebhard 1969, p. 78). Looking at S&M scenes may, for example, give us some insight into how fantasies are produced and shared, the nature of the relationship between fantasy and sexuality, and the connection between play and sexual behavior.

The S&M world is a secret world. It has been described as a "velvet underground." Andreas Spengler (1977) noted that secrecy is one of the special norms of sadomasochists. Thus, a study of such behavior may help to reveal the nature of secrecy as a social phenomenon. The conditions under which secrets are developed, shared, kept, and revealed, and the functions of secrecy for social groups are important topics. We do know that different S&M worlds vary in the importance of secrecy to their participants and in the degree to which, and in the conditions under which, they make themselves visible. The gay "leathersex" subculture is much more visible than the heterosexual S&M world. Most large cities have gay S&M bars; with few exceptions, the contacts of heterosexual S&Mers are limited to private, small networks. The question is, why should this be the case? Are stigmatized groups such as homosexuals more tolerant of other sorts of unconventional sexual behavior? Is it that gays who are already "out" have (or feel that they have) less to lose by revealing sadomasochistic needs than do heterosexuals? Or is the explanation for the greater visibility of gay S&M that it occurs within an already existing structure and is therefore an easily accepted variation on a theme? Contacts among gay S&Mers seem to be more easily made in part because there are many more non-S&M settings in which people can find partners who may be willing to try an S&M scene as an extension of sex play.

Much sadomasochistic activity occurs in dyads and triads. Thus, studying S&M is likely to add to our knowledge of the ways in which small groups operate. How, for example, are decisions reached? How do people place limits on their behavior and that of others? What happens when these norms are violated?

What is the connection between small S&M groups and the larger S&M world? How do people discover this world, get integrated into it, and develop contacts with potential partners? How do their identities, motives, and behavior develop and change over time? These and many other questions are answered by the articles that we have collected in this volume.

Finally, one good reason for studying sadomasochistic behavior is that it may be more prevalent in the larger society than one might suspect. Writers like Judith Coburn (1977) claim that there is a growing "S&M chic" in this country.

Sadomasochistic themes appear more and more in advertising, books, and movies. Adult sex toy shops and boutiques are becoming more and more prevalent. Even in 1969, Gebhard noted that

> The prevalence of unconscious sadomasochism is impossible to ascertain, but it must be large if one can make inferences from book and magazine sales and from box office reports. We do know that consciously recognized sexual arousal from sadomasochistic stimuli are not rare. The Institute for Sex Research found that one in eight females and one in five males were aroused by sadomasochistic stories. . . . (p. 79)

All of the articles in this collection focus on sadomasochism as a form of social behavior. This means that these studies concern themselves with the interaction *between* individuals situated within a subcultural context. While they examine sadomasochism from a variety of viewpoints, all of the writers share some basic assumptions about S&M behavior. Without losing sight of the individual as participant, they are all concerned with the production and dissemination of social meanings as a central part of the sadomasochistic world. Their essays refrain from making the kinds of moral judgments often contaminating the work of earlier scholars.

In one way or another, each of the contributions to this book addresses the issues first outlined in the Gebhard article. They have been organized into three sections reflecting specific levels of analysis. The first section, "Selves," is concerned with the individual within the S&M milieu. The second section, "Scenes," focuses primarily upon the subcultural aspects of S&M. The third section, "Structures," discusses the organizational features of the sadomasochistic experience.

References

Breslow, N., L. Evans, and J. Langley. 1985. "On the Prevalence and Roles of Females in the Sadomasochistic Subculture: Report on an Empirical Study." *Archives of Sexual Behavior* 14: 303–17.

Caprio, Frank S. 1955. *Variations in Sexual Behavior.* New York: Grove.

Coburn, Judith. 1977. "S&M." *New Times* 8 (February 4): 43–50.

Ellis, Havelock. 1942. *Studies in the Psychology of Sex,* vol. 1, part 5. New York: Random House.

Freud, Sigmund. 1938. *The Basic Writings of Sigmund Freud,* trans. and ed. A. A. Brill. New York: Modern Library.

Gebhard, Paul H. 1969. "Fetishism and Sadomasochism," pp. 71–80 in *Dynamics of Deviant Sexuality,* ed. Jules H. Masserman. New York: Grune & Stratton.

Kamel, G. W. Levi. 1980. "Leathersex: Meaningful Aspects of Gay Sadomasochism." *Deviant Behavior* 1: 171–91.

Krafft-Ebing, R. von. 1965. *Psychopathia Sexualis,* trans. Franklin S. Klaf. New York: Stein and Day.

Moser, Charles, and Eugene E. Levitt. 1977. "An Exploratory-Descriptive Study of a Sadomasochistically Oriented Sample." *Journal of Sex Research* 23: 322–37.

Spengler, Andreas. 1977. "Manifest Sadomasochism of Males: Results of an Empirical Study." *Archives of Sexual Behavior* 6: 441–56.

Stekel, Wilhelm. 1965. *Sadism and Masochism.* New York: Grove Press.

Weinberg, Thomas S. 1978. "Sadism and Masochism: Sociological Perspectives." *Bulletin of the American Academy of Psychiatry and the Law* 6: 284–95.

Weinberg, Thomas S., and Gerhard Falk. 1980. "The Social Organization of Sadism and Masochism." *Deviant Behavior* 1: 379–93.

Richard von Krafft-Ebing

Psychopathia Sexualis

Sadism: Association of Active Cruelty and Violence with Lust

Sadism, especially in its rudimentary manifestations, seems to be of common occurrence in the domain of sexual perversion. Sadism is the experience of sexual [*sic*] pleasurable sensations (including orgasm) produced by acts of cruelty, bodily punishment afflicted on one's own person or when witnessed in others, be they animals or human beings. It may also consist of an innate desire to humiliate, hurt, wound, or even destroy others in order thereby to create sexual pleasure in one's self.

Thus it will happen that one of the consorts in sexual heat will strike, bite, or pinch the other, that kissing degenerates into biting. Lovers and young married couples are fond of teasing each other, they wrestle together "just for fun," indulge in all sorts of horseplay. The transition from these atavistic manifestations, which no doubt belong to the sphere of physiological sexuality, to the most monstrous acts of destruction of the consort's life can be readily traced.

Where the husband forces the wife by menaces and other violent means to the conjugal act, we can no longer describe such as a normal physiological manifestation, but must ascribe it to sadistic impulses. It seems probable that this sadistic force is developed by the natural shyness and modesty of women towards the aggressive manners of the male, especially during the earlier periods of married life and particularly where the husband is hypersexual. Woman no doubt derives pleasure from her innate coyness and the final victory of man affords her intense and refined gratification. Hence the frequent recurrence of these little love comedies. . . .

In the civilized man of today, in so far as he is untainted, associations between lust and cruelty are found, but in a weak and rather rudimentary degree. If such therefore occur and in fact even light atrocious manifestations thereof, they must be attributed to distorted dispositions (sexual and motoric spheres).

They are due to an awakening of latent psychical dispositions, occasioned by external circumstances which in no way affect the normal individual. They are not accidental deviations of sentiment or instinct in the sense as given by the modern doctrine of association. Sadistic sensations may often be traced back to early childhood and exist during a period of life when their revival can by no manner of means be attributed to external impressions, much less to sexual temper.

Sadism must, therefore, like Masochism and the antipathic sexual instinct, be counted among the primitive anomalies of the sexual life. It is a disturbance (a deviation) in the evolution of psychosexual processes sprouting from the soil of psychical degeneration.

That lust and cruelty often occur together is a fact that has long been recognized and is frequently observed. Writers of all kinds have called attention to this phenomenon. . . .

In an attempt to explain the association of lust and cruelty, it

is necessary to return to a consideration of the quasi-physiolog-
ical cases, in which, at the moment of most intense lust, very ex-
citable individuals, who are otherwise normal, commit such acts
as biting and scratching, which are usually due to anger. It must
further be remembered that love and anger are not only the most
intense emotions, but also the only two forms of robust emotion.
Both seek their object, try to possess themselves of it, and naturally exhaust themselves in a physical effect on it; both throw the
psycho-motor sphere into the most intense excitement, and thus,
by means of this excitation, reach their normal expression.

From this standpoint it is clear how lust impels to acts that
otherwise are expressive of anger. The one, like the other, is a
state of exaltation, an intense excitation of the entire psycho-
motor sphere. Thus there arises an impulse to react on the object
that induces the stimulus, in every possible way, and with the
greatest intensity. Just as maniacal exaltation easily passes to
raging destructiveness, so exaltation of the sexual emotion often
induces an impulse to spend itself in senseless and apparently
harmful acts. To a certain extent these are psychical accompani-
ments; but it is not simply an unconscious excitation of innerva-
tion of muscles (which also sometimes occurs as blind violence);
it is a true hyperbole, a desire to exert the utmost possible effect
upon the individual giving rise to the stimulus. The most intense
means, however, is the infliction of pain.

Through such cases of infliction of pain during the most
intense emotion of lust, we approach the cases in which a real
injury, wound, or death is inflicted on the victim. In these cases
the impulse to cruelty which may accompany the emotion of
lust, becomes unbounded in a psychopathic individual; and, at
the same time, owing to defect of moral feeling, all normal
inhibitory ideas are absent or weakened.

Such monstrous, sadistic acts have, however, in men, in
whom they are much more frequent than in women, another
source in physiological conditions. In the intercourse of the
sexes, the active or aggressive role belongs to man; woman
remains passive, defensive. It affords man great pleasure to win

a woman, to conquer her; and in the art of love making, the modesty of woman, who keeps herself on the defensive until the moment of surrender, is an element of great psychological significance and importance. Under normal conditions man meets obstacles which it is his part to overcome, and for which nature has given him an aggressive character. This aggressive character, however, under pathological conditions may likewise be excessively developed, and express itself in an impulse to subdue absolutely the object of desire, even to destroy or kill it.

If both these constituent elements occur together—the abnormally intensified impulse to a violent reaction toward the object of the stimulus, and the abnormally intensified desire to conquer the woman—then the most violent outbreaks of sadism occur.

Sadism is thus nothing else than an excessive and monstrous pathological intensification of phenomena—possible, too, in normal conditions in rudimental forms—which accompany the psychical sexual life, particularly in males. It is of course not at all necessary, and not even the rule, that the sadistic individual should be conscious of his instinct. What he feels is, as a rule, only the impulse to cruel and violent treatment of the opposite sex, and the coloring of the idea of such acts with lustful feelings. Thus arises a powerful impulse to commit the imagined deeds. In as far as the actual motives of this instinct are not comprehended by the individual, the sadistic acts have the character of impulsive deeds.

When the association of lust and cruelty is present, not only does the lustful emotion awaken the impulse to cruelty, but *vice versa*; cruel ideas and acts of cruelty cause sexual excitement, and in this way are used by perverse individuals.

Masochism: The Association of Passively Endured Cruelty and Violence with Lust

Masochism is the opposite of sadism. While the latter is the desire to cause pain and use force, the former is the wish to suffer pain and be subjected to force.

By masochism I understand a peculiar perversion of the psychical sexual life in which the individual affected, in sexual feeling and thought, is controlled by the idea of being completely and unconditionally subject to the will of a person of the opposite sex; of being treated by this person as by a master, humiliated and abused. This idea is colored by lustful feeling; the masochist lives in fantasies, in which he creates situations of this kind and often attempts to realize them. By this perversion his sexual instinct is often made more or less insensible to the normal charms of the opposite sex—incapable of a normal sexual life—psychically impotent. But this psychical impotence does not in any way depend upon a horror of the opposite sex, but upon the fact that the perverse instinct finds an adequate satisfaction differing from the normal—in woman, to be sure, but not in coitus.

But cases also occur in which with the perverse impulse there is still some sensibility to normal stimuli, and intercourse under normal conditions takes place. In other cases the impotence is not purely psychical, but physical, i.e., spinal; for this perversion, like almost all other perversions of the sexual instinct, is developed only on the basis of a psychopathic and, for the most part, hereditarily tainted individuality; and as a rule such individuals are given to excesses, particularly masturbation, to which the difficulty of attaining what their fancy creates drives them again and again.

I feel justified in calling this sexual anomaly "Masochism," because the author *Sacher-Masoch* frequently made this perversion, which up to his time was quite unknown to the scientific world as such, the substratum of his writings. I followed thereby the scientific formation of the term "Daltonism," from *Dalton*, the discoverer of color-blindness.

During recent years facts have been advanced which prove that Sacher-Masoch was not only the poet of Masochism, but that he himself was afflicted with this anomaly. Although these proofs were communicated to me without restriction, I refrain from giving them to the public. I refute the accusation that I have coupled the name of a revered author with a perversion of the sexual instinct, which has been made against me by some admirers of the author and by some critics of my book. As a man Sacher-Masoch cannot lose anything in the estimation of his cultured fellow-beings simply because he was afflicted with an anomaly of his sexual feelings. As an author he suffered severe injury so far as the influence and intrinsic merit of his work is concerned, for so long and whenever he eliminated his perversion from his literary efforts, he was a gifted writer, and as such would have achieved real greatness had he been actuated by normal sexual feelings. In this respect he is a remarkable example of the powerful influence exercised by the sexual life—be it in the good or evil sense—over the formation and direction of man's mind.

The number of cases of undoubted masochism thus far observed is very large. Whether masochism occurs associated with normal sexual instincts, or exclusively controls the individual; whether or not, and to what extent, the individual subject to this perversion strives to realize his peculiar fancies; whether or not, he has thus more or less diminished his virility—depends upon the degree of intensity of the perversion in the single case, upon the strength of the opposing ethical and aesthetic motives, and the relative power of the physical and mental organization of the affected individual. From the psychopathic point of view, the essential and common element in all these cases is *the fact that the sexual instinct is directed to ideas of subjugation and abuse by the opposite sex.*

Whatever has been said with reference to the impulsive character (indistinctness of motive) of the resulting acts and with reference to the original (congenital) nature of the perversion in sadism, is also true in masochism.

In masochism there is a gradation of the acts from the most repulsive and monstrous to the silliest, regulated by the degree of intensity of the perverse instinct and the power of the remnants of moral and aesthetic countermotives. The extreme consequences of masochism, however, are checked by the instinct of self-preservation, and therefore murder and serious injury, which may be committed in sadistic excitement, have here in reality, so far as known, no passive equivalent. But the perverse desires of masochistic individuals may in imagination attain these extreme consequences.

Moreover, the acts to which masochists resort are in some cases performed in connection with coitus, i.e., as preparatory measures; in others, as substitutes for coitus when this is impossible. This, too, depends only upon the condition of sexual power, which has been diminished for the most part physically and mentally by the activity of the sexual ideas in the perverse direction, and not upon the nature of the act itself.

Sigmund Freud

Sadism and Masochism

The tendency to cause pain to the sexual object and its opposite, the most frequent and most significant of all perversions, was designated in its two forms by Krafft-Ebing as sadism for the active form, and masochism for the passive form. Other authors prefer the narrower term, *algolagnia,* which emphasizes the pleasure in pain and cruelty, whereas the terms selected by Krafft-Ebing place the pleasure secured in all kinds of humility and submission in the foreground.

The roots of active algolagnia, sadism, can be readily demonstrable in the normal individual. The sexuality of most men shows an admixture of aggression, of a desire to subdue, the biological significance of which lies in the necessity for overcoming the resistance of the sexual object by actions other than mere *courting.* Sadism would then correspond to an aggressive component of the sexual instinct which has become independent and exaggerated and has been brought to the foreground by displacement.

The concept of sadism fluctuates in everyday speech from a

Excerpted from Sigmund Freud, *The Basic Writings of Sigmund Freud,* ed. and trans. A. A. Brill. New York: The Modern Library (1938), pp. 569–71.

mere active or impetuous attitude toward the sexual object to an absolute attachment of the gratification to the subjection and maltreatment of the object. Strictly speaking, only the last extreme case can claim the name of perversion.

Similarly, the designation masochism comprises all passive attitudes to the sexual life and to the sexual object: in its most extreme form the gratification is connected with suffering of physical or mental pain at the hands of the sexual object. Masochism as a perversion seems further removed from the normal sexual goal than its opposite. It may even be doubted whether it ever is primary and whether it does not more often originate through transformation from sadism.[1] It can often be recognized that masochism is nothing but a continuation of sadism directed against one's own person in which the latter at first takes the place of the sexual object. Clinical analysis of extreme cases of masochistic perversions show that there is a cooperation of a large series of factors which exaggerate and fix the original passive sexual attitude (castration complex, guilt).

The pain which is here overcome ranks with the loathing and shame which are the resistances opposed to the libido.

Sadism and masochism occupy a special place in the perversions, for the contrast of activity and passivity lying at their bases belong to the common traits of the sexual life.

That cruelty and the sexual instinct are most intimately connected is beyond doubt taught by the history of civilization, but in the explanation of this connection no one has gone beyond the accentuation of the aggressive factors of the libido. The aggression which is mixed with the sexual instinct is, according to some authors, a remnant of cannibalistic lust—that is, a participation of the domination apparatus, which serves also for the gratification of the other ontogenetically older great need.[2] It has also been claimed that every pain contains in itself the possibility of a pleasurable sensation. Let us be satisfied with the impression that the explanation given concerning this perversion is by no means satisfactory and that it is possible that many psychic strivings unite herein into one effect.[3]

The most striking peculiarity of this perversion lies in the fact that its active and passive forms are regularly encountered together in the same person. He who experiences pleasure by causing pain to others in sexual relations is also capable of experiencing pain in sexual relations as pleasure. A sadist is simultaneously a masochist, though either the active or the passive side of the perversion may be more strongly developed in him and thus, represent his preponderant sexual activity.[4]

We, thus, see that certain perverted tendencies regularly appear in contrasting pairs, which . . . is of great theoretical value. It is furthermore clear that the existence of the contrast, sadism and masochism, can not readily be attributed to the mixture of aggression. On the other hand, one may be tempted to connect each synchronously existing contrast with the united contrast of male and female in bi-sexuality, the significance of which is reduced in psychoanalysis to the contrast of activity and passivity.

Notes

1. Later reflections which can be supported by definite evidence concerning the structure of the mental systems and of the activities of instincts therein, have changed my judgment concerning masochism very widely. I have been led to recognize a primary erotogenic masochism from which there develops two later forms, a feminine and a moral masochism. Through a turning back of an unconsumed sadism directed against oneself during life there arises a secondary masochism which is added to the primary masochism. (See Freud, Das ökonomische Problem des Masochisten, Int. Zeit. f. Psa, 10, 121, 1924. Translated into English in *Collected Papers*, vol. 2, p. 255. Hogarth Press.)

2. Cf. here the later studies on the pregenital phases of the sexual development, in which this view is confirmed.

3. From the researches just cited, the contrasted pair, sadism-masochism, originates from a special source of impulses and is to be differentiated from the other "perversions."

4. Instead of substantiating this statement by many examples, I will merely cite Havelock Ellis (*The Sexual Impulse*, 1903): "All known cases of sadism and masochism even those cited by Krafft-Ebing always show (as has already been shown by Colin, Scott, and Fere) traces of both groups of manifestations in the same individual."

Havelock Ellis

Studies in the Psychology of Sex

In the foregoing rapid survey of the great group of manifestations in which the sexual emotions come into intimate relationship with pain, it has become fairly clear that the ordinary division between "sadism" and "masochism," convenient as these terms may be, had a very slight correspondence with facts. Sadism and masochism may be regarded as complementary emotional states; they cannot be regarded as opposed states. Even de Sade himself, we have seen, can scarcely be regarded as a pure sadist. A passage in one of his works expressing regret that sadistic feeling is rare among women, as well as his definite recognition of the fact that the suffering of pain may call forth voluptuous emotions, shows that he was not insensitive to the

Excerpted from Havelock Ellis, *Studies in the Psychology of Sex,* Volume III, *Analysis of the Sexual Impulse, Love and Pain, The Sexual Impulse in Women,* Second Edition, Revised and Enlarged, Philadelphia: F. A. Davis Company, 1926: pp. 159–60, 166, 171–72, 175–76. This 1926 version of Ellis's work is a reissue of the 1913 revised and expanded second edition. The first edition was originally published in 1903. Reprinted by permission of Professor François Lafitte, trustee of the Havelock Ellis Estate.

37

charms of masochistic experience, and it is evident that a merely bloodthirsty vampire, sane or insane, could never have
retained, as de Sade retained, the undying devotion of two
women so superior in heart and intelligence as his wife and sis-
ter-in-law. . . . It is clear that, apart from the organically morbid
twist by which he obtained sexual satisfaction in his partner's
pain—a craving which was, for the most part, only gratified in
imaginary visions developed to an inhuman extent under the
influence of solitude—de Sade was simply to those who knew
him, "*un aimable mauvais sujet*" gifted with exceptional intellectual powers. Unless we realize this we run the risk of confound-
ing de Sade and his like with men of whom Judge Jeffreys was
the sinister type.

It is necessary to emphasize this point because there can be no
doubt that de Sade is really a typical instance of the group of perversions he represents, and when we understand that it is pain
only, and not cruelty, that is the essential in this group of manifestations we begin to come nearer to their explanation. The
masochist desires to experience pain, but he generally desires
that it should be inflicted in love; the sadist desires to inflict pain,
but in some cases, if not in most, he desires that it should be felt
as love. How far de Sade consciously desired that the pain he
sought to inflict should be felt as pleasure it may not now be possible to discover, except by indirect inference, but the confessions
of sadists show that such a desire is quite commonly essential. . . .

We have thus to recognize that sadism by no means involves
any love of inflicting pain outside the sphere of sexual emotion,
and is even compatible with a high degree of general tender-
heartedness. We have also to recognize that even within the sexual sphere the sadist by no means wishes to exclude the victim's
pleasure, and may even regard that pleasure as essential to his
own satisfaction. We have, further, to recognize that, in view of
the close connection between sadism and masochism, it is highly probable that in some cases the sadist is really a disguised
masochist and enjoys his victim's pain because he identifies himself with that pain.

But there is a further group of cases, and a very important group, on account of the light it throws on the essential nature of these phenomena, and that is the group in which the thought or the spectacle of pain acts as a sexual stimulant, without the subject identifying himself clearly either with the inflicter or the sufferer of the pain. Such cases are sometimes classed as sadistic; but this is incorrect, for they might just as truly be called masochistic. The term algolagnia might properly be applied to them (and Eulenburg now classes them as "ideal algolagnia"), for they reveal an undifferentiated connection between sexual excitement and pain not developed into either active or passive participation. Such feelings may arise sporadically in persons in whom no sadistic or masochistic perversion can be said to exist, though they usually appear in individuals of neurotic temperament. . . .

We have seen that the distinction between "sadism" and "masochism" cannot be maintained; not only was even de Sade himself something of a masochist and Sacher-Masoch something of a sadist, but between these two extreme groups of phenomena there is a central group in which the algolagnia is neither active nor passive. "Sadism" and "masochism" are simply convenient clinical terms for classes of manifestations which quite commonly occur in the same person. We have further found that—as might have been anticipated in view of the foregoing result—it is scarcely correct to use the word "cruelty" in connection with the phenomena we have been considering. The persons who experience these impulses usually show no love of cruelty outside the sphere of sexual emotion; they may even be very intolerant of cruelty. Even when their sexual impulses come into play they may still desire to secure the pleasure of the persons who arouse their sexual emotions, even though it may not be often true that those who desire to inflict pain at these moments identify themselves with the feelings of those on whom they inflict it. We have thus seen that when we take a comprehensive survey of all these phenomena a somewhat general formula will alone cover them. Our conclusion so far must be that under certain abnormal circumstances pain, more especially the mental representation of pain, acts as a powerful sexual stimulant.

The reader, however, who has followed the discussion to this point will be prepared to take the next and final step in our discussion and to reach a more definite conclusion. The question naturally arises: by what process does pain or its mental representation thus act as a sexual stimulant? The answer has over and over again been suggested by the facts brought forward in this study. Pain acts as a sexual stimulant because it is the most powerful of all methods for arousing emotion. . . .

In the ordinary healthy organism, however, although the stimulants of strong emotion may be vaguely pleasurable, they do not have more than a general action on the sexual sphere, nor are they required for the due action of the sexual mechanism. But in a slightly abnormal organism—whether the anomaly is due to a congenital neuropathic condition, or to a possibly acquired neurasthenic condition, or merely to the physiological inadequacy of childhood or old age—the balance of nervous energy is less favorable for the adequate play of the ordinary energies in courtship. The sexual impulse is itself usually weaker, even when, as often happens, its irritability assumes the fallacious appearance of strength. It has become unusually sensitive to unusual stimuli and also, it is possible—perhaps as a result of those conditions—more liable to atavistic manifestations. An organism in this state becomes peculiarly apt to seize on the automatic sources of energy generated by emotion. The parched sexual instinct greedily drinks up and absorbs the force it obtains by applying abnormal stimuli to its emotional apparatus. It becomes largely, if not solely, dependent on the energy thus secured. The abnormal organism in this respect may become as dependent on anger or fear, and for the same reason, as in other respects it may become dependent on alcohol.

Paul H. Gebhard

Sadomasochism

Sadomasochism may be operationally defined as obtaining sexual arousal through receiving or giving physical or mental pain. Unlike fetishism, analogues are common among other mammalian species wherein coitus is preceded by behavior which under other circumstances would be interpreted as combative. Temporary phases of actual fighting may be interspread in such precoital activity. In some species, such as mink, sexual activity not infrequently results in considerable wounds. This precoital activity has definite neurophysiological value in establishing, or reinforcing, many of the physiological concomitants of sexual arousal such as increased pulse and blood pressure, hyperventilation, and muscular tension. Indeed one may elicit sexual behavior in some animals by exciting them with nonsexual stimuli. This may explain why sadomasochism is used as a crutch by

Excerpted from Paul H. Gebhard, "Fetishism and Sadomaso-chism," pp. 71–80 in Jules Masserman, M.D., ed., *Dynamics of Deviant Sexuality: Scientific Proceedings of the American Academy of Psychoanalysis*, New York: Grune & Stratton, 1969. Reprinted by permission of Grune & Stratton and the Kinsey Institute for Research in Sex, Gender & Reproduction, Inc., as well as the author.

aging men in our society who require some extra impetus to achieve arousal. From a phylogenetic viewpoint it is no surprise to find sadomasochism in human beings.

Sadomasochism is embedded in our culture since our culture operates on the basis of dominance-submission relationships, and aggression is socially valued. Even our gender relationships have been formulated in a framework conducive to sado-masochism: the male is supposed to be dominant and aggressive sexually and the female reluctant or submissive. Violence and sex are commingled to make a profitable package to sell through the mass media. This is no innovation—for centuries the masochistic damsel in distress has been victimized by the evil sadist who is finally defeated by the hero through violent means.

Relatively few sadomasochists are exclusively sadists or exclusively masochists; there is generally a mixture with one aspect predominant. This mixing is sometimes necessitated by circumstances: sexual partners are extremely difficult to find and consequently, for example, if two masochists meet they are obliged to take turns at the sadist role. This role-taking is made easier by ability to project. The masochist playing the sadist may fantasy himself receiving the pain he is inflicting.

Sadists are far rarer than masochists, and female sadists are so highly prized that masochists will travel hundreds of miles to meet them. I postulate that this imbalance between sadists and masochists is a product of our culture wherein physical violence, particularly to someone of the opposite gender, is taboo and pro-ductive of intense guilt. To strike is sin; to be struck is guiltless or even virtuous in a martyrdom sense. Even more psychody-namically important is masochism as an expiation for the sin of sexuality. During childhood, puberty, and part of adolescence sexual behavior is punished and it is easy to form an association between sexual pleasure and punishment. The masochist has a nice guilt relieving system—he gets his punishment simultane-ously with his sexual pleasure or else is entitled to his pleasure by first enduring the punishment.

It is important to realize that pain *per se* is not attractive to the masochist, and generally not to the sadist, unless it occurs in an arranged situation. Accidental pain is not perceived as pleasurable or sexual. The average sadomasochistic session is usually scripted: the masochist must allegedly have done something meriting punishment, there must be threats and suspense before the punishment is meted out, etc. Often the phenomenon reminds one of a planned ritual or theatrical production. Indeed, sadomasochistic prostitutes often report their clients give them specialized instructions to follow. Genet's *Balcony* is true to life. When one appreciates this one realizes that often in the relationship the sadist is not truly in charge—the sadist is merely servicing the masochist. The sadist must develop an extraordinary perceptiveness to know when to continue, despite cries and protests, and when to cease. A sadist who goes too far or stops prematurely may find his ineptitude has cost him a sexual partner. Not infrequently sadomasochistic activity is interspersed with loving and tenderness. This alternation makes the process far more powerful. Police and brainwashers use the same technique of alternate brutality and sympathy to break their subjects.

Sadomasochism is extremely complex. Some achieve orgasm during the pain; in other cases the sadomasochism only constitutes the foreplay and the session culminates in conventional sexual behavior. Some masochists dislike the pain while it is being inflicted, but obtain gratification by anticipation of the pain or by thinking about it after it has ceased. Lastly, there are the bondage people who do not enjoy pain but are stimulated by constraint, mild discomfort, and a sense of helplessness. Bondage has both sadistic and masochistic aspects. The sadist has the pleasure of rendering his partner helpless and at his mercy—a favorite sexual theme in mythology, literature, and fantasy. The masochist bondage enthusiast enjoys not only the restraint itself but the guilt relieving knowledge that if anything sexual occurs it is not his or her fault. Also as Dr. Douglas Alcorn points out, some persons derive a sense of comfort and security from physical constraint. Lastly, the hood, often used in bondage, offers the advantage of depersonalization and heightens the helplessness through interfering with sight, hearing, and vocalization.

Both sadomasochism and bondage are often replete with fetish items including specialized clothing and restraint or torture devices. All this offers the devotee substantial additional gratification. The average heterosexual or homosexual has relatively little paraphernalia for supplementary pleasure and it offers scant opportunity for ingenuity or creativity.

The prevalence of unconscious sadomasochism is impossible to ascertain, but it must be large if one can make inferences from book and magazine sales and from box office reports. We do know that consciously recognized sexual arousal from sadomasochistic stimuli are not rare. The Institute for Sex Research found that about one in eight females and one in five males were aroused by sadomasochistic stories, and roughly half of both sexes were aroused by being bitten.

The etiology of sadomasochism, while the subject of much writing especially in the form of interminable German books, is not well understood. In individual cases the genesis may be clear as psychoanalysis and psychiatry amply demonstrates, but these individualistic explanations do not suffice for the phenomenon as a whole. After all, the supply of English headmasters and Austrian girl friends is limited. We must turn to broad hypotheses, and I will offer a rather simplistic one.

First, we may assume on the basis of mammalian studies and history that we humans have built-in aggressive tendencies. Second, it is equally clear that males are on the whole more aggressive than females. Experiments indicate this is in large part an endocrine matter: androgens elicit or enhance aggression. Thirdly, animal and human social organization is generally based on a dominance-submissiveness relationship, a peck-order. Fourthly, when one couples the difficulties of sexual gratification with the problems involved in living in a peck-order society, one has an endless source of frustration which lends itself to expression in pathological combinations of sex and violence. Note that in our own culture when we wish to say that someone was badly victimized we use sexual terms such as, "he got screwed." From a rational viewpoint we should apply the words "he got screwed" to someone who had had a pleasurable experience, but we have unfortunately mixed sex with dominance-submissiveness behavior.

This using sex as a symbol brings up the puzzle as to why explicitly sexual sadomasochism, like fetishism, seems the monopoly of well-developed civilizations. One never hears of an aged Polynesian having to be flogged to obtain an erection, and for all their torture and bloodshed there seem to have been no de Sades amongst the Plains Indians or Aztecs. While it is true that in various preliterate societies sexual activity often involves moderate scratching and biting, well-developed sadomasochism as a lifestyle is conspicuous by its absence. It may be that a society must be extremely complex and heavily reliant upon symbolism before the inescapable repressions and frustrations of life in such a society can be expressed symbolically in sadomasochism. Sadomasochism is beautifully suited to symbolism: what better proof of power and status is there than inflicting humiliation or pain upon someone who does not retaliate? And what better proof of love is there than enduring or even seeking such treatment?

Reference

Alcorn, Douglas: Personal communication.

SELVES
S&M IDENTITIES

Introduction

G. W. Levi Kamel's "The Leather Career: On Becoming a Sadomasochist" describes in detail the stages in identity formation for gay male sadomasochists. Kamel examines the acquisition of a "leatherman" identity as a dynamic process involving attempts at "sense-making" on the part of men entering the S&M world. Kamel illustrates the interplay between what one observes and how one interprets and applies this information.

The next selection, "Autobiography of a Dominatrix," is included to provide a description of one pathway into S&M. Juliette follows an uncharted path into S&M. She learns about sadomasochism through "sense-making," redefining as desirable each step of the way into S&M. Juliette identifies herself primarily as a prostitute. Thus, she reports having been amazed when she met a woman who was involved in S&M "on her own time."

Kamel and Weinberg illustrate the diversity in S&M and show that participation in this behavior is part of a social process by viewing involvement in sadomasochism as a "career." They adopt this perspective from Erving Goffman, who has noted that people who share similar "stigmas" tend to have much the same experiences and come to view themselves and others in similar ways. In the presentation of a number of S&M biographies and in their discussion, it is made clear that becoming a sado-masochist is to a large extent part of an interactive process. Those who have recognized their sadomasochistic feelings must seek out others who share their desires. Then they must learn how to construct and control S&M scenes. Through socialization, they learn specific norms and values. Other people, who have not previously recognized any sadomasochistic interests, become involved in S&M through a variety of relationships.

Moser and Levitt describe the demographic characteristics, sexual behavior, and self-perceptions of a self-defined sample of 178 men and 47 women. They provide evidence that people come into the S&M world relatively late and learn to accept themselves and their identity with few problems. They find their behavior satisfying and do not see it as shameful. Many members of the sadomasochistic world also tend to be "versatile" or "switchable," willing to take both dominant or submissive roles, rather than being exclusively one or the other.

G. W. Levi Kamel

The Leather Career: On Becoming a Sadomasochist

If little is known about the origins of homosexual and hetero-sexual feelings in human beings, probably less is known about the emergence of sadomasochistic desires. This ignorance is not the result of a lack of interest in this phenomenon. On the contrary, the writings of many of the greatest sexologists and personality theorists contain speculations about sadomasochism.

One of the first such works was authored by the nineteenth-century neuropsychiatrist, Richard von Krafft-Ebing, for whom sadomasochism held an intense fascination. In *Psychopathia Sexualis,* his most popular book, first published in the 1880s, he identified the psychology of women as a primary source of sado-masochistic impulses. Specifically, he suggested that sadism in males was probably "developed by the natural shyness and modesty of woman toward the aggressive manners of the male . . . particularly where the husband is hypersexual." In other

This paper is a revised version of parts of "Leathersex: Meaningful Aspects of Gay Sadomasochism," which originally appeared in *Deviant Behavior: An Interdisciplinary Journal* 1: 171–91, 1980. An edited version of the remainder of that article appears in the section on "Structures" in the present volume. Reprinted by permission of the author.

words, sadistic desires develop in oversexed men who court sexually or emotionally distant women. Krafft-Ebing further wrote that, "the facts of masochism are certainly among the most interesting in the domain of psychopathology . . . (masochism) represents a pathological degeneration of the distinctive psychical peculiarities of woman." Here he says that masochism originates from a sort of frenzied female psyche. Yet, Krafft-Ebing's speculations do not explain sadomasochism without the female influence, as with gay male S&M.

In his early writings, Sigmund Freud also considered sadomasochism to be a pathology. Years later, however, he refined his thinking on the topic. He came to view sadistic tendencies as an extension of the pleasure principle, an understandable, if extreme, instance of the sexual urge. Masochism, on the other hand, which seemed to confuse Freud more than sadism, was explained as a tendency toward self-destructiveness. Even in their final form, however, Freud's theories have left us with many unanswered questions about the nature of sadomasochism.

Not all of the older ideas about sadomasochism were cast in such negative terms as those used by Krafft-Ebing and Freud. Havelock Ellis, for example, who recognized his own sadomasochistic interests, suggested that such desires might be traced to the play habits of sensitive children. He saw S&M as an outlet for atavistic impulses; one which left the individual more inclined toward tenderness in everyday life.

Perhaps the least negative approach to an explanation of S&M comes from the writings of Kinsey's colleague, Paul H. Gebhard. Dr. Gebhard, an anthropologist, believed sadomasochism to be a cultural phenomenon. That is, it has its origin in the norms and values of the larger social environment, rather than being an expression of idiosyncratic individual pathology. In his classic article on the subject, "Fetishism and Sadomasochism," Gebhard asserts the following:

> Sadomasochism is embedded in our culture since our culture operates on the basis of dominance-submission relationships, and aggression is socially valued. Even our gender relation-

ships have been formulated in a framework conducive to sado-masochism: the male is supposed to be dominant and aggressive sexually and the female reluctant or submissive.

Gebhard continues his criticism, pointing a finger at media images that fuse sex and violence on the one hand, and perpetuate stereotypical sex roles on the other. Thus, Gebhard presents a purely cultural theory of the origin of sadomasochism. The problem with this theory, and with the others mentioned here, is that they only try to explain how S&M desires develop. They say nothing at all about how people become S&M practitioners, how they become involved with the S&M society, and how they come to form an S&M identity.

In order to explain these social-psychological events, we will be using the concept of "career." By "career" we mean a sequence of stages or steps along a path, with each career step suggesting a new level of involvement in leathersex and a new stage in the development of a leather identity. There are at least six such steps, which we have called "disenchantment," "depression," "curiosity," "attraction," "drifting," and "limiting."

Disenchantment

It is not unusual for younger, less experienced gay men to become somewhat disenchanted with the gay world a few years after coming out. This disenchantment may have any number of sources: the difficulty in forming a permanent relationship; frustrating experiences with overpossessive companions; the seeming insincerity, coldness, and shallowness of many bar games; or simple boredom with flashing disco lights, pretty faces, and excessive sex. This sense of disappointment with gay community night life is often intensified if hetero-culture norms (such as "monogamy-ideal" or "sex-means-love") are transplanted into the erotic reality of the homosexual male. These norms seldom work well in the context of all-male sexuality.

The most frequent complaint among disillusioned newcomers is that the average bar-going gay man is simply not "macho" enough to be attractive. The "straight" world conceptions of masculinity, usually ranging from the beer-drinking butch image to the overweight biker, often linger in the minds of those who are new to the gay scene. The more relaxed masculinity and manners of many gay men seem less erotic when compared with the hypermasculine milieu of the straight world. Newcomers sense this disparity more deeply than other gay men, often leading them to a second step toward leathersex, a time of depression.

Depression

During the depression period, some gay men experience isolation anew—a second "closet." They often leave gay night life behind, returning to earlier days of loneliness and a fantasy sex life.

This depression may last from a few months to a few years, with different degrees of severity. Lasting periods of depression are typically marked by sexual outlets not traditionally part of the gay club and night life. Such outlets may include truck stop and tearoom encounters, adult bookstore and movie house pickups, sex ad liaisons, and adventures with hustlers.

Commonly, the age at which gay men enter this second closet, if they do at all, is the middle to late twenties, depending upon when involvement in the gay community first began. Further, most of those who experience a second closet eventually reenter the gay world with more appropriate expectations; but some others do not. For some men, the second closet is a period of psychological preparation for another facet of the homosexual experience, the world of leather. This preparation involves movement to yet a third step, that of curiosity.

Curiosity

The gay man in his second closet, unlike the man in his first, has a working knowledge of the gay subculture. He knows the rules of interaction; where clubs, taverns, and organizations are located; and how he may participate. He is also wiser about his sexual orientation and his consequent position in society at large. Many of the anxieties he was forced to grow with, such as the belief that he must be the only homosexual in town, have since disappeared. In his second closet, he is aware of what he is missing.

The leather scene, however, like other minority elements of the gay community, may still be mysterious to him. It is likely that he knows only the stereotypes about S&M, as they may have been introduced to him by some of his first gay acquaintances. Such stereotypes of leathersex label it "emotionally distant," "sexually immature," "physically dangerous," and "preoccupied with hypermasculinity," all misguided perceptions of sadomasochism.

The stigma of exaggerated masculinity may lead some discouraged gay men to become curious about the S&M scene and to wonder whether a compatible partner might be found among the ranks of the leather clique.

Increasing curiosity often encourages a person to seek out more information about leathersex. Avenues of such information may include perusals through both pornographic and non-pornographic periodicals; questioning friends; weighing hearsay, myths, and rumors; and visiting leather-oriented establishments. The latter may include out-of-town visits to S&M bath houses. As the search progresses, many individuals decide that leathersex is not what they want after all. They will find other alternatives for sexual expression, or drop out of intimate relations altogether. For many others who explore their S&M potential, an attraction may begin to develop.

Attraction

As a man becomes attracted to leathersex, he may be laying the foundation upon which to construct an S&M self. That is, he may begin to believe that personal involvement in leathersex is at least plausible, and that he *could* be a participant if he wanted to. During the attraction stage, the perception that leathersex is within the bounds of one's erotic possibilities is crucial to the inception of an S&M identity. S&M activities must be conceivable before they can be seen as a part of the self.

This may also be a stage of growing excitement and anticipation about some future rendezvous with leathersex, when the individual might experience some physical and emotional contact. Social interaction often increases during this time, as does one's repository of knowledge about S&M. There may also be some contemplation about such rules-of-the-game as "limits," "signals," and other agreed upon safety devices. One discovers that leathermen have mutual respect for each other, and this information usually reduces fears of physical or emotional harm.

It is common for those men who become attracted to leathersex to be in their late twenties or early thirties, although this is far from a hard and fast rule. This stage involves a type of second coming-out phase, when leather bars, baths, and perhaps bike organizations become a focal point of attention. Feelings of depression often diminish at this time, yielding to a growing drift into leathersex.

Drifting

Near the beginning of the drifting stage the novice commits himself to finding an S&M partner. He decides to experiment with leathersex. The search for an initial partner may be carried out in many ways, but probably the most common way is to increase visits to leather bars and baths. The diversity and variety of the leather crowd gives the person a chance to cruise for a compatible partner who is willing to train him.

Finding someone who will teach a beginner the ropes may not be so easy. One of the first discoveries a novice may make is that S&M experience is considered an asset among many leathermen; personality, youth, or good looks alone will not usually attract a mate. An initial encounter might therefore require an exchange of relative youth or good looks for senior "know how."

Leathersex requires by its nature a certain amount of acting ability. A successful (i.e., satisfying) encounter depends very much on the capacity of the participants to sustain each other's erotic fantasies. Inexperienced men are sometimes not aware of this unwritten rule, and seem interested only in their own sexual satisfaction. They have not yet fully appreciated the vital psychological link between their desires and those of their partner. This requirement of interdependence for psychosexual fulfillment is something better apprehended only after a number of S&M episodes have occurred. To experienced leathermen, rookies often appear unable to feign the appropriate leathersex attitudes in order to set aside their own needs and to satisfy the erotic requirements of their partner. This is why newcomers are so often viewed as selfish, both during and after leather scenarios.

Inexperience in developing and sustaining mutually satisfactory scenarios may also help to explain why the novice tends to prefer the role of the bottom. As slave, the beginner is able to enter S&M scenes more easily because he is supposedly led by his master into the various activities that make up the drama. His script is prescribed for him. After some period of drift in sexual slavery, the bottom usually decides that he too would like to lead. It is perhaps this decision, combined with learning the nuts-and-bolts of "what masters do," that allows the slave to begin taking the role of the top. The bottom-to-top path, as most leather enthusiasts know, is typical of the S&M career.

The period of drift is probably the longest period of all. It is actually a cluster of phases in which the leatherman makes a "new sense" of each activity in which he engages. It is a period during which previously uninteresting sexual behaviors gradually become a part of his erotic desires. As drift into sophisticated leather practices continues, the individual finds himself enjoying sexual practices once thought to be meaningless or silly.

During this drifting and sense-making process, a leather identity emerges. The person begins to see himself as a part of the S&M scene. He feels as though he is a member of a particular group of men. No longer a novice or a newcomer, he is more in control of the sexual situations in which he becomes involved. He is now ready for many more S&M encounters.

Drifting is often the step in a leather career in which new relationships with other gay men develop. The person may prefer a pattern of casual sex with a series of mates, or settle into a monogamous relationship. He may go through cycles of greater or lesser sexual interest and involvement. Whatever his preferences, he eventually reaches the final step of limiting.

Limiting

A person enters the limiting stage when he experiments with one or more erotic acts and chooses not to make a new sense of them, those he perhaps wishes he had not tried. Instead of being able to assign feelings of pleasure to these behaviors, he experiences some anxiety. While drifting he is, of course, in a process of expanding his limits, not yet certain about the boundaries of his S&M tastes. During the limiting period, however, he practices leathersex with more or less full awareness of what he will and will not enjoy.

The leathermen who reach the limiting stage in their S&M careers are perhaps the most sexually satisfied (and satisfying) of all. They have defined the boundaries of their sexuality, and they are most likely to appreciate the needs and limits of others. With a fuller understanding of S&M, experienced leathermen often are better equipped to use good judgment during hot and heavy encounters.

The range of erotic variations in leathersex is probably greater than many gay people suspect. This makes limiting even more important in S&M. Failure to limit might prove unpleasant. Leather society has an elaborate system of spoken and unspoken social rules, dos and don'ts that govern the action of its members. Limiting underlies many of these rules.

Conclusions

The six-stage career framework used here does not apply to every sadomasochist. In fact, it probably fits well for only a very few. To suggest otherwise would be to disregard one of the most fascinating aspects of the leather world—the wide variations of actors and scripts. However, among many leathermen these steps are remarkably typical, representing the various stages that seem to be important in becoming a sadomasochist.

The S&M reality is sometimes thought to be a negative facet of the gay community, a thorn in the side of liberation. S&M is sometimes viewed as inconsistent with the ideology of the present generation of gay people, which holds that homosexuality is, and ought to be, the love of one's own sex in its pure, natural, and most beautiful form. Just as this view shuns playing daddy (pederasty), playing favors (prostitution), or playing lady (cross-dressing), it also refuses to sanction playing roles (sadomasochism). Sadomasochists not only voluntarily adopt roles, they overstate them, something gays often see as a heterosexist problem. Still, S&M is a topic about which most gay people are at least willing to talk. This is usually not true among heterosexuals. It is perhaps this relative degree of openness that explains why leathersex is practiced within a context of social rules and norms, and why it does not involve any real violence, coercion, or human abuse. Heterosexual culture, by contrast, does not readily tolerate open discussion about sadomasochism. Indeed, most heterosexuals probably do not know much about what it is, whether they harbor such feelings or not.

References

Gebhard, Paul H. 1969. "Fetishism and Sadomasochism," pp. 71–80 in *Dynamics of Deviant Sexuality*, ed. Jules H. Masserman. New York: Grune and Stratton.

Krafft-Ebing, Richard von. 1965. *Psychopathia Sexualis*, trans. Franklin S. Klaf. New York: Stein and Day.

Juliette

Autobiography of a Dominatrix

It was 1968. Young people were claiming a new type of inde-
pendence and completely shunning the customs and morals of
the older generation. Everybody seemed to be getting involved
and experimenting. I was only seventeen years old, restless, and
curious about it all. I wanted to be involved and involved I got.

I had my bags packed for a year before I left for New York
City. I left with a girl friend the day after our high school graduation ceremonies. I can still remember my mother driving us to the
airport that morning, all the time warning me about the perils of
the big city. But I just laughed at her, because what did she know
about life anyhow? Besides, it would be different for me. I would
have a good life, and I was a big girl now and could take care of
myself. I had twelve hundred dollars in my pocket when we
arrived. This was supposed to tide me over until I could find
some type of employment. We stayed with a friend we had met
that Easter when we came down to the city to spend the weekend.
He was a photographer and an antique dealer and wanted to get
my friend involved in modeling. She was a truly beautiful girl, the

---

Specially written for this volume.

kind that you see on the cover of *Seventeen* magazine. Everybody made a fuss over her and told her how great she was. By the end of the month she was working as a photographic model and meeting just the right people. It was just like in a storybook. I, on the other hand, was always in her shadow. Nobody even noticed that I was alive. Besides, I was overweight and this made me even more despondent, unhappy, and extremely jealous. I wanted to be popular and have men notice me like they did her.

The nights were exciting in the city, and I was meeting people in clubs that I had only seen on the TV and heard on records. It was about this time that I really got involved in the whole drug subculture. It was through a woman that I met at a club one night. She was a groupie who would sleep with anybody who was in a group, or with any man for that matter. We got an apartment together on the city's Lower East Side right next to the Electric Circus and around the corner from the Fillmore East. My friend seemed to know about everything and she knew everyone in the Village. On Friday and Saturday nights her friends would come in from Brooklyn and the Bronx to go to the Circus but would first stop by our house and shoot up. We used to call them weekend junkies. These were people who would only get high once a week or so just for kicks. I had no say about what was going on in the apartment, it was like she had complete control over me. I just went along with anything she said.

She would always coax me to try dope. "I just want you to feel the rush," she would say to me, "and if you sit still you won't get sick." So one night I finally consented. I can remember that night as if it were yesterday. I put out my right arm, closed my eyes, and let the sweet juices of Miss Heroin flow into my veins. She was right. The rush was fantastic and I sat very still and didn't get sick. This was to be the beginning of a very long love affair with the White Lady. I started to shoot up pretty regularly then and my money was soon gone. But never fear because my friend was here. She knew two guys who would give us $25 apiece if we would just go to bed with them. I didn't want to do it, but once again she talked me into it. I found out that it wasn't all that bad. We took the money that we made and didn't pay the rent, but instead we spent it on getting high. We soon lost the apartment and went our separate ways.

I was alone with nowhere to go and no money in my pocket. For weeks I drifted from place to place and only rested when I could find an apartment to crash at. I was so scared and was getting sick from not eating and never resting. . . .Back out on the streets again, I met a man and we hooked up together and started selling heroin. The dope we had was good, and before you knew it we had a booming business and I had a habit as long as my arm—a dealer's habit. We made lots and lots of money and shot lots and lots of dope. I was secure once again. This sense of security didn't last for very long however, because after a few months of heavy dealing we finally got busted. The only thing left to do in order to survive and to keep a hole in my arm was to start turning tricks.

I really didn't know anything about the business at that time because I had only done it once before. But I was a trooper and quickly learned the ways of the "ho" stroll.[1] I really didn't have any choice because I was now a bona fide junkie and had a dealer's habit besides. The area that I started on was E. 14th Street, the armpit of prostitution. Eighty percent of the girls who worked that area were junkies. Most of the tricks that were turned were done in cars—quick blow jobs. Home for me now had become the Valentine Hotel. This was the sort of place that girls turned tricks in and where welfare people and derelicts lived. The decor of the place wasn't anything you'd see in *Better Homes and Gardens* magazine. It smelled, but so did I. The people on the streets never bothered me much, because I always stayed to myself, trying to make myself invisible to the pimps and especially to the police. There was never any time to sleep because you had to find the money for your next fix. That was all that was important. The only time you got to relax was if you made a big sting.[2] Then you would just get a room and shoot up until the money was gone and you had to start the whole process all over again.

One night, while I was walking the streets looking for someone to pick up, I ran into this guy who told me that he was an ex-cop and asked me if I would be interested in working in a house with a Madam. I looked pretty dirty and grubby and couldn't understand what he wanted with me. He said if I wanted to, he would take me over that night to meet this woman, so I went. She lived in this beautiful apartment building with a doorman and the whole bit. We went inside, and I was introduced to a rather plump woman about twenty-five years old. She explained to me that her business was all done through a book with numbers that she had accumulated over the years and some that she had bought from a Madam who was going out of business and getting married. She said that the tricks started at an average of $25 and up. I would keep half of everything I made and half went to her for setting up the date. This sounded great and I wouldn't have to be on the streets any longer.

I went to work for her the next day and made about a hundred and fifty dollars. It was easy; all the appointments were set up for me, and the Johns[3] were all real nice. But unlike working on the streets, I had to learn to take my time with the Johns and to be more generous with my body. Everything was working out good and I had stopped shooting dope and was buying Methadone on the street so I could function better. But all this time I'm working, I'm thinking how I can get hold of that book and just make all the money for myself instead of giving her half. I took a lot of money from her but never got the book.

From there I went on to work at other houses that had a different system of getting their tricks. I started to work for a man and his wife who started the business so they could pay off old gambling debts. It was sort of an arrangement that he had made with the people that he owed the money to. This house was set up in a brownstone. They rented the whole place and used all three floors. There were four girls who worked at a time. There were two women there who just answered telephones, and one who would answer the door and introduce the available girls. They got their business by placing ads in *Screw* magazine. Each girl was given a fictitious name and an article was run every week in the paper about how luscious she was and what her specialties were. Specialities ranged from French, Greek, and TV sessions to bondage.[4] The sessions ran for about forty minutes and that included anything you wanted for as many times as you wanted. The rooms were big and beautiful and with real wood-burning fireplaces in every room.

The first day I worked there I had on a halter top and a pair of hot pants. I thought for sure that this would certainly attract some attention. My first trick was a priest. He was a regular at this place and was easy to take care of, all he wanted was a blow job and ran out after it was over like a scared rabbit. I went back downstairs after I was finished and just sat and watched as everybody got picked except me. Then this very nice-looking man came in and chose me. We went upstairs and went through the preliminaries and then I asked him what type of session he wanted. He told me that he picked me because of the hot pants that I was wearing. He said that he had been in a Nazi concentration camp as a child and that a woman in charge there had worn shorts and high boots like the ones that I had on. He was a sort of servant to this woman and she would make him clean her boots. She would do this by making him sit in a chair and then take the heel of her boot and grind it into his crotch. He said that even as a child this used to arouse him and now it was something that he had to have done to him at least once a month. This was the first time I had ever encountered this type of freaky request. And so I stood over him while he [lay] on the floor and ground my feet into his crotch. Other than this, his sex life was quite normal according to him, but he just had an obsession with this particular act. Most of the sessions I had while working at this house were mostly straight, mainly because they had no type of equipment to work with. But the few men who did come in and ask for special sessions gave me my initial knowledge of sadomasochism.

I worked in this place for about six months until I got fired because I was falling asleep on the customers, and they started to complain to the management. I was turning an average of fifteen tricks a day. This meant that my take-home pay every night was about $300. As soon as I got out of work I would catch a cab, and go down and see the drug pusher.

When I left this place I knew that I couldn't work the streets anymore, it just wasn't the same. So I got myself a job at another house. This was a specialty house that dealt mostly in various kinds of S&M sessions. This house was set up in the ground apartment of a huge complex. All the sessions were $75 apiece. It was a wonderland for the man who had exotic tastes in sex. We had every type of device imaginable to make you as uncomfortable as we possibly could. There were, to mention a few: whips, paddles, cat-o'-nine-tails, chains, leather binders, leather blindfolds, handcuffs, rope, stiletto shoes, nurses' outfits, enemas, suspension equipment, nipple clippers, penis stretchers, dildos of every imaginable shape and size, and vibrators. It was also fun to make up your own types of tortures. It was incredible the things you could do with just a simple pair of tweezers and a candle stick. But not every man liked to be physically tortured. Some of these gentlemen just preferred to be verbally humiliated, or spanked with just your hand while you told them how naughty they were. But let us not forget the man who enjoys golden showers or to be defecated on. The average person might think that men who enjoy this type of perverted sex must be monsters. On the contrary, they were mostly professional people like lawyers, doctors, executives, or people in the arts. It wasn't bad working these kinds of sessions. I mean, God, anything was better than flatbacking and having to be mauled and pulled at all day long. Besides, by this time I was pretty hardened and I enjoyed beating and humiliating men who had done the same to me. And when I got into a session I would put every ounce of strength I had into it. I hated all of these bastards: No matter how nice they were, they were still all just tricks to me, and disgusting. There was the fat man with club feet who would come to see me every week just so I could tell him how disgusting and repulsive he was, for which he always gave me a big tip. And there was a nice German gentleman who came to see me once a week to have his fanny beaten with a hair brush.

He would take off all of his clothes and go hide in the bathroom and I would pretend I was his older sister and discovered him doing something naughty. He would act just like a small child and say, "I didn't do nothin'." I would pretend to get mad at him for lying to me, grab him and throw him over my knee and beat him with the brush until his whole ass was just one big red welt. This man also always gave me a good tip.

Men who are into things like role-playing usually pay very well when they can find a pro who's a good actress and who knows what she's doing. It's very important to be as realistic as possible. Sometimes they like you to dress up for these sessions. This was really popular with people who liked enemas. The whole thing of seeing a sadistic nurse in her little uniform while she makes a man take in all the water from a two-quart enema bag is just the biggest turn-on in the world for some people. Then there were the men who were leather worshippers and just adored seeing a woman dressed in a black leather jumpsuit and high heel leather boots. They would get very excited just touching the leather and loved to take their tongues and lick your boots all over. It's funny the way the most ridiculous things can turn some people on. Some people would want a session that they had never tried before just because it sounded like it might be exciting in their mind's eye. But once they actually do it, it's a whole other ball game. Sometimes, thinking about a perverted act can be much more exciting than the act itself.

We also advertised out of *Screw,* but we would put pictures of the girls in the ads. This place was in full swing for about eight months, at which time I managed the house and collected the money from the girls and paid them at the end of the night. One day, someone in one of the other apartments got wind that there was a house of ill repute in the building, and the whole neighborhood was in a panic. They had petitions that they were passing around the block for the people to sign to get us out of the building. They constantly harassed us and said that they were being attacked by the customers who came to see us. Well, we finally had to close the place down because it was impossible to work there any longer; so then everyone had to look for new employment. I looked through the trade papers and found an ad where they were looking for girls for a strictly outgoing service. I met a young man who had heard about what happened at the other place I was working at and he told me about this man who was looking for someone to run a house for him and to be his partner. I would not have to make any kind of investment, and the apartment and phones would be provided for me. He would be a silent partner and all he wanted was his share of the money every month. This seemed too good to be true. I told him the experience that I had and that I had owned several of my own houses before, which was a lie. But, damn, I had accumulated enough knowledge by now to run ten houses. He dropped off the keys to the apartment the next day; we moved in the house and prepared for the grand opening of "Cosmopolitan Playgirls."

We placed only one large ad in the paper. Basically, it stated that we were an outgoing service and would travel to any of the boroughs, including New Jersey, and, of course, that we specialized in discipline. Business was really slow for the first couple of weeks; there was only myself and another girl working, and one driver. The driver knew a woman who was a nurse and who was interested in working. I talked to her on the phone and we made a date for her to come down so I could interview her. She was super! She walked into the apartment wearing a full length mink coat with a studded dog collar around her neck, and she carried a whip made out of a horse's tail. When she took off her coat she had on a black leather halter top, shorts, and black leather boots with reinforced iron fronts for kicking better. She loved S&M not only for the money, but she also did it on her own time. When I told her that we were only charging $50 an hour she said that she refused to work for so little money, and I should have a starting price of at least $100 an hour plus the driver's fee. I told her that she was crazy, that there wasn't an ad in the paper that was charging over $65 now. She said that I could easily get that much money and got on the phone and set up my first $100 date. I learned that I could charge astronomical prices if I had the right girls, a good sales pitch, and, of course, tons of equipment.

The business started to grow, and before you knew it I had ten girls working for me, two phone girls, and five drivers. All the girls who were working for me had never worked in a house before. I had a college girl, a nurse, a housewife, a professional model, and a woman who worked in the kitchen of a famous hotel, all part-time working girls. These girls were not hardened by the streets or pimps and rather enjoyed what they did. The tricks loved it, and all the girls were beautiful and, most important, every one was happy and making big bucks. After the business got in full swing, we upped our prices for the S&M sessions and just had the straight sessions at $100. I completely stopped working now and just took care of the management part of the business. I felt like a queen, like I had finally made it. We started to entertain such people as foreign ambassadors, and my girls were escorts for many important business clients who wanted to entertain associates. The money was coming in like crazy and just as fast as it came in I spent it on drugs and clothes. My environment had changed and so had my standard of living, but I hadn't changed at all. I now had the opportunity to make something of myself and save some money, but I didn't. Even the girls were getting disgusted with me and started leaving. It finally ended with me getting arrested for promoting prostitution. I'll never know to this day how it happened, except that one of the girls who worked for me dropped a dime.[5] I left New York after that, got on a Methadone program, and came back home after eight long and hard years of hustling.

I'm drug-free now and physically okay, but I still yearn for the excitement of the business and that secure feeling I had when I was high. I don't know if I'll make it in your world but I've never tried so hard in my life. So I'm just gonna keep on truckin' and maybe I'll succeed, or maybe I'll die.

Notes

1. "Ho" stroll is the vicinity where prostitutes congregate to meet customers.

2. "Sting" refers to getting money by cheating someone.

3. "Johns" are the customers of prostitutes.

4. "French" refers to oral-genital sex; "Greek" is anal sex; "TV" is the term for transvestism; and "bondage" is the tying up of a person.

5. "Dropped a dime": called the police.

G. W. Levi Kamel
and Thomas S. Weinberg

Diversity in Sadomasochism:
Four S&M Careers

The S&M world is a diverse subculture. Most probably it would not be inaccurate to say that there are a number of different S&M subcultures, or, perhaps, sub-subcultures. There are variations not only in terms of basic sexual orientations such as heterosexual and homosexual with many possibilities for blendings and crossings over, but there are also individuals and, consequently, social groups with tastes for various kinds of costumes and behaviors. There are, for instance, numerous gay leather and motorcycle clubs. People who are "into" transvestism, enemas, urination ("golden showers" or "watersports"), defecation ("scat" or "brown showers"), whips, bondage, and the like can all find not only partners, but also newsletters, magazines, and clubs catering to their specific preferences.

The variety of sadomasochistic identities and behaviors makes the study of S&M both fascinating and challenging. S&M "careers"[1] can be studied as a social as well as a psychological phenomenon. That is, instead of making the individual as "patient" the sole focus of interest, as is done traditionally in

---

Specially written for this volume.

clinical case studies, we can treat the individual as a *social actor* and examine his behavior from *his* perspective. We are especially interested in his definitions of situations, the ways in which he applies *socially acquired* meanings to situations and learns to make sense of what is going on through a process of socialization to sadomasochism. Our focus here is very definitely on social interaction and the ways in which meanings are learned and shared as much as it is on the individual actor.

The following examples illustrate not only the endless varieties of career paths along which S&Mers travel, but they also point out the importance of other persons in teaching both behaviors and attitudes toward sadomasochism as a form of erotic expression. The nature of S&M as a collaborative event is obvious in all of these histories. For example, we can see how Jeanie is socialized by Daniel and the ways in which she has learned to accommodate herself to his needs. She has even come to define sadomasochist acts as pleasurable and erotically stimulating. Glen's career illustrates how an individual's perceptions and goals may change as a result of the learning experiences he has had with other S&M devotees. It also shows how S&M couples can segregate their sadomasochistic behavior from other areas of their relationship. Robbie's story points out the importance of mutual respect and affection for people involved in ongoing S&M relationships. Implicit in his history is that there are norms governing sadomasochistic interaction and that control is shared by both partners. Vito has not yet settled upon a relatively fixed sexual identity. We can see in his history the dynamic nature of S&M careers through the ways in which he tries to make sense of his feelings by experimenting with female prostitutes and male sexual partners.

Daniel and Jeanie: An S&M Relationship

Sadomasochism is perhaps best understood as an interactive phenomenon. It is above all a cognitive event that emerges as

sadist and masochist confront each other. One way to understand S&M, therefore, is to take a look at relationships that are
based heavily on the extremes in dominance and submission.
Daniel, twenty-seven, and Jeanie, twenty-six, are one couple
who practice sadomasochism. Married three years, Daniel and
Jeanie have formed a strong S&M bond, which permeates their
sexual life and their everyday activities. Their relationship began
at a relatively early period in their lives, when Daniel was a
sophomore in high school. A brief profile of Daniel and Jeanie as
individuals is instructive before describing their life together.

Daniel has been interested in sadomasochism since he can
remember. As a child, his daydreams took him on a number of
mental excursions into masochism. He describes one of them:

> I used to fantasize things like getting cornered by a bunch of
> girls on the playground and getting peed on just for fun.
> Sometimes I would think about getting tied up by them first. I
> was about twelve or fourteen then. . . . Oh yes, I would get
> erections with those thoughts, but I can't say how the thoughts
> started with me.

Later, Daniel recalls, his masochistic fantasies became more
sexually explicit in nature. With remarkable clarity and detail,
Daniel remembers,

> I would think about being tortured by two tall black women.
> I'd be in their apartment in the ghetto and they would accuse
> me of stealing their money. I took the money from their purs-
> es. They were dressed a little differently each time I thought of
> them, but always they had leather straps under their clothes,
> high heeled black boots, and steel toes. Usually I thought
> about them whipping me. They would strip me and torture
> my cock. They would sit on me and force me to perform oral
> sex on them. Just before the session was over they would give
> me permission to jack off.

It is often the case among male heterosexual sadomasochists
that transvestic activities hold some erotic meaning. The mean-

ing may be transsexual—the desire actually to be female—or it may signify humiliation, an important feeling for most masochists. In the latter situation, cross-dressing activities are fetishistic. That is, they involve sexual foreplay and orgasm. Daniel is no exception. Dressing at least partly in female attire has been a part of his erotic adventures since puberty. Beginning at the age of twelve or so, and until his late teens, Daniel used many of his mother's clothes for masturbation. Articles such as shoes, panties, brassieres, and nylon stockings were among his favorites (although he also enjoyed donning his mother's robes when he was alone at home). Later, he substituted his wife's wardrobe, as he presently does. Daniel reports that his cross-dressing adventures have always had a high degree of erotic content, and that shame and humiliation are feelings that emerge *during* (rather than after) these episodes. His cross-dressing increases as opportunity allows and when other sexual activities are less frequent.

Unlike Daniel's sadomasochistic desires, Jeanie's did not develop until adulthood and marriage. She, in fact, sees such feelings as an outgrowth of her relationship with Daniel. She insists they were not a part of her childhood. In her words:

> Dan got me into S&M. Now I like it a lot. I never realized how much I could get into it but I sure do. Of course my feelings about Daniel helped. I love him. . . . At first I was confused and repulsed, but underneath I knew I had the potential for S&M in me.

Jeanie relates that she has recently come to prefer the masochistic role with Daniel, although that was not always the case. It was a "switch" in Daniel's preference that probably generated her own change. Although she is not fully aware of how the switch occurred with Daniel, she recognizes its importance for the present S&M arrangement between Daniel and herself.

In the absence of his wife, Daniel openly provides his account of how the change from masochist to sadist occurred in his mental life. Shortly after his marriage to Jeanie, Daniel found his masochistic desires increasingly difficult to suppress. Fearful of his new bride's negative reaction to the suggestion that they experiment with sadomasochism, Daniel began developing a relationship with a female co-worker who seemed promising:

> Brenda seemed like the type who would go for it. She dominated conversations and was hard and sometimes mannish acting. She was cold but attractive, and hardly seemed naive about sex with men. I was sure she could get into dominating me, so I started an affair with her as soon as I got the chance.

Within the context of a series of clandestine encounters with his new mistress, Daniel gradually introduced sadomasochistic activities. He made attempts to persuade her to dominate him in several ways: with bondage, watersports, the administration of pain, and other S&M related practices. His mistress

> just didn't have the heart for it. She surprised me, 'cause she wasn't the dominant type as I thought she would be. But I didn't give up, because something told me S&M was in her head somewhere.

As a final attempt, Daniel consciously decided to teach Brenda S&M dominance by demonstration. He himself practiced dominant sexual techniques on her:

> I started out easy, like with pinching her nipples. I spanked her a little, then I got tougher, screwing her as hard as I could. Then I got into humiliating her verbally, calling her a slut while I fucked her.

To Daniel's amazement, Brenda enjoyed these sessions more than she had any previous encounters. To his even greater amazement, Daniel discovered that he, too, was enjoying these S&M scenes. Along with his increasing pleasures as a master, their relationship grew stronger over a period of about two years. Daniel's affair was so intense that it began to interfere with his marriage. At this point, Daniel broke off the affair with Brenda. He describes this break:

It was getting to be too much. I wasn't falling in love with her, but she was fulfilling my S&M needs so much. Actually, she was fulfilling my need to dominate, which I didn't even know I had until I started with her. I was growing dependent on her emotionally. It was starting to hurt my marriage and even my job. It was taking too much time too, so I broke it off. By that time she was a real slave and I was a real master. Her submission fed my dominance and vice versa 'till it got to the point where little else occupied my head.

After his final meeting with Brenda, Daniel entered a period of erotic suppression. He held S&M desires and feelings at bay, spending more time and energy with his wife. Daniel found this arrangement satisfying for some time. Then, slowly at first, his S&M desires returned. This time, however, these desires were primarily dominant rather than submissive. His fantasies went in wild new directions, exploding into his mind's eye as never before. This switch in preference he attributes to his previous affair with Brenda:

By bringing out the bottom (masochist) in Brenda, I found out how great being a top (sadist) could be. She brought out my dominance at the same time. . . . Yeah, I guess I have a core-like slave in me, but being master turns me on too . . . especially with my wife now.

Presently, Daniel and Jeanie are discovering sadomasochism as never before. At the very beginning of their marriage, Jeanie unenthusiastically played the role of "top" in mild S&M scenes. Now, she finds far greater pleasure as a "bottom." Daniel also finds the new arrangement to his liking:

I'm getting her into being strongly dominated now and she responds beautifully. It's so beautiful that she amazes me with every encounter. It's terrific being married to someone who turns me on so intensely.

Daniel and Jeanie do not feel they have yet reached their limits in sadomasochism, but believe that the intensity of their feelings for each other will guide them safely to those limits. Sadomasochistic desires in the relationship between Daniel and Jeanie developed to their present state through a series of phases, beginning with marriage, the experimentation with Daniel as slave early in their marriage, Daniel's secret sexual episodes with Brenda, and finally with his dominance over his wife. As an indirect consequence of Daniel's lifelong sadomasochistic desires, his wife Jeanie eventually found and developed her own. These desires in adulthood thus emerged as a result of their emotional and erotic correspondence.

Glen: Profile of a Typical Gay S&Mer

Glen is not a particularly remarkable man in appearance, standing five-feet-seven-inches and weighing 150 pounds. He has rather handsome features, and is of masculine manner. Even his occupation as inventory clerk for a large northeastern manufacturer, and his midwestern, middle-class background are not remarkable. What makes Glen different from others in his cohort is his homosexuality, and his interests in sadomasochism.

From the time Glen was five years old, he remembers having a sense of isolation from other members of his family. With his mother, he recalls, relations were distant. Glen was continually attempting to gain his mother's attention, but the struggle to make ends meet forced her to help her husband in his trade. Little time or energy was left to spend with Glen; but even the few moments shared with his mother were cool. Throughout his formative years, Glen recalls:

> My mother seldom had much time for me. She never looked me in the eyes or held me close like I wanted. She was always with my father who was a furniture refinisher. She usually did the shit-work he didn't want to do, like staining wood. She seemed to do the dirty work so willingly, but hardly spoke to me when I came around.

Interaction with his father was even less satisfactory for young Glen. Although he was normally considered a hard worker and good provider for his family, Glen's father experienced periods of drunkenness and violent behavior. These periods were marked by episodes of beatings and family life disruptions. According to Glen:

> All the time I was growing up, until I was twelve or thirteen, I was afraid of my father and his violent temper. Everyone in the family was afraid of him, but people outside the family figured he was a great guy. Outwardly he was fine, but when he was alone with his wife and us kids, he was hell. . . . We never knew when the violence would erupt, and there seemed to be no way to control it. We just waited in fear and anticipation of his arrival.

Glen recalls having several psychologically painful experiences with his father as well. These were generally characterized by hostility and an attempt to humiliate Glen. His father was especially cruel toward Glen's effeminacy. From a very early age, Glen was the object of such derogatory name-calling as "Daddy's sissy" and "the family faggot." One particularly memorable occasion occurred when Glen accompanied his father to a major-league baseball game:

> I remember when I was ten, my father took me to a baseball game, something I always hated. I was bored to death, not caring about what I was watching. I tried not to show it by talking about the game like I was interested. I really liked it that he was taking me somewhere, and I didn't want him to stop doing that. Without thinking about his reaction, I blurted out something about how awful I thought it was that the players were trampling the beautiful grass in the outfield. I asked my father why they had to play on the grass; and with a look of disgust, he asked me in a low voice if I knew what a faggot was. I said no, knowing that whatever it was, it was bad, and I must be one of them. I felt very odd and very much alone.

A profound feeling of being different stayed with Glen throughout his early years. This feeling was reinforced by two brothers who, Glen admits, usually wanted little to do with him, and by his sister, who avoided him entirely. Peers, too, played with him only long enough to mock him and oust him from his childhood activities. But it was not until later, when Glen was fifteen or so, that he came to realize the root cause of his feelings and manners. It was at that age that Glen found himself intensely attracted to a male classmate.

Glen's realization that he was homosexual led him to isolate himself from the outside world even more. While finishing high school, he concentrated on study and on his part-time job. Then, on the evening of his graduation from high school, Glen left his home and family behind. He took up residence in a western state, and continued to battle his homosexuality for several years.

In an attempt to defeat his homosexuality, Glen married at the age of twenty-three. But during three years of marriage, his attraction toward other males only intensified. At the same time that his wife began appealing to him for cooperation in starting a family, Glen finally realized that his homosexual feelings would not cease so easily. His divorce followed shortly after this realization. He then "came out" as openly gay to his family, admitting his homosexuality.

Glen was now twenty-five. Thus far sadomasochism had not been a part of Glen's homosexual feelings in any identifiable way. Other than fleeting adolescent erotic fantasies of bondage and constraint during sexual intercourse with another man, Glen had never thought about sadism and masochism.

S&M slowly entered Glen's sexual life. His first years of gay life were marked by rather conventional sexual activities. The newness and excitement of cruising and promiscuity precluded anything so sophisticated as sadomasochism. But the newness did not last.

S&M was always available to Glen during his initial experiences in the gay world. There were plenty of friends and acquaintances who were involved in S&M to some degree, and he knew where to find the local leather set. Glen first began patronizing leather bars in order to find masculine partners for sex. Many of the gay men he found in other bars were simply not masculine enough for him. Then, Glen explains,

> I suddenly got out of gay life. Somehow it suddenly seemed cold and cruel, superficial and dishonest. I was depressed and wanted nothing to do with sex for a while. This lasted for a year or so. I guess I just got burned out. . . . It wasn't turning me on anymore. . . . Something was lacking.

Glen later began searching for that "something" among the S&M enthusiasts who frequented leather bars. As his curiosity about S&M developed, Glen began asking himself questions such as which role he would be happiest with, who would train him in S&M practices, and what his reactions would be. His curiosity soon led to a series of initial encounters with a new friend named Bill who:

> taught me to be a slave and I loved it. It seemed so right for me that I felt I had come home for the first time in my life. Serving him gave me the warmest feelings I had ever had with anyone. It was great.

Since his first encounters with Bill and others, Glen has most often preferred the passive (insertee or "bottom") role. This preference has taken many forms during sadomasochistic scenarios, including slave and master, prisoner and warden (with a variation involving punk and wolf[2]), and even innocent hitchhiker and dirty old man.

As his experiences with sadomasochistic sex have accumulated, the goals and meanings of such encounters have changed. Initially they were opportunities for sexual self-discovery. They served to "break the ice" and to eliminate any residual guilt concerning his atypical sexual leanings. They helped to shape his sexuality as well, both defining and discovering what he found to be pleasurable. On this matter, Glen noted that "it is impossible to say whether these scenes were erotic because they somehow expressed feelings I already had, or whether they actually created the feelings in the first place."

Gradually, however, Glen came to find fulfillment in those encounters which helped him discover the sexuality of his partners. It was this newer practice of satisfying the needs of others that perhaps accounts for Glen's emerging need to have a permanent S&M relationship. Glen describes this need as he first felt it:

> I found myself wanting someone to call my own after a few years of this . . . in S&M. I wanted someone special. I guess I wanted to be a slave to someone forever. I knew it was supposed to be hard for two men to have a lasting relationship, but I wanted to try.

After several attempts to form a lasting relationship, Glen met his present lover, Jim. Jim is extremely dominant, Glen explains, but loving and, above all, caring. Glen has now spent the last four years as a slave to Jim, a period he describes as very satisfying:

> The last four years with Jim have been great. I've never felt so close to anyone in my life. We are able to communicate about everything, and his dominance over me has not become a way for him to take advantage, as it did with others. There are almost no jealousy trips and I feel 100 percent his. We are super in love.

The master and slave roles are generally confined to the bedroom. There is virtually no spillover into other areas of their relationship. Domestic decisions, chores, and responsibilities are shared equally. S&M roles, however, are almost never exchanged between Glen and Jim. Jim is always master. To have it otherwise, Glen explains, would disrupt the "fragile balance." That is, switching S&M roles would tend to destroy the images each has of the other, and thereby diffuse the auras of dominance and submission. For most S&M relationships, this diffusion is popularly thought to send shock waves throughout the delicate web of master-slave interaction. Both sexual and nonsexual arrangements would become problematic; they would again be strangers to each other's ways, yet they would have the added burden of a number of previously established expectations about each other's behavior. Like most other S&M couples, Glen and Jim have found it desirable to maintain their respective sex roles while dispensing with them in other areas of their domestic life.

Robbie: A Masochistic Bisexual

Robbie is twenty-three years old. He is the second of six children. When he was seven or eight years old, his father left home. Robbie has not seen him since then. He was raised by his mother, with whom he feels especially close. He also reports feeling very close to his brothers and sisters.

Robbie remembers having been very unhappy during late grammar school. He was harassed by the other children at his parochial school; they labeled him a "faggot." At the time, he did not know what the word meant. In retrospect, Robbie thinks he might have been effeminate at that age, but he does not remember having noticed any feminine traits in himself. This was a very painful time. "When I was young," he says, "I put myself in a shell. I had the feeling of being an outcast for a very long time." By his teens this seems to have changed, and Robbie says that he was happy as a teenager and fairly popular in high school. He attributes this later acceptance by his peers to their maturity and the development of more liberal attitudes.

Robbie's first sexual experience, at the age of sixteen, was with a man in his late twenties who had offered him a ride home from a concert. Robbie says that he enjoyed this encounter, but subsequent same-sex experiences were very infrequent during high school years.

At the age of seventeen, Robbie had his first sexual experience with a woman who was a few years older than him. After this initial exposure to heterosexual relations, he began having sex on a regular basis with other women.

Robbie defines himself as bisexual, since he enjoys having sex with both men and women. Lately, though, he has been more sexually active with male partners. Despite having had some same-sex experiences in his late teens, Robbie claims that he has not been very attracted to men until relatively recently:

> I knew I'd go to bed with both sexes. One interesting thing is that I really did not look at men lustfully. Gay porno didn't turn me on. Straight porno did and still does . . . and then I look at gay porno and only if it's well done in some ways aesthetically or maybe being kinky too, I may get turned on.

Robbie is a masochist. Ever since early childhood, he has had masochistic fantasies. Some of his thoughts are rather unusual. For example, in addition to having had both male- and female-oriented S&M fantasies with himself as the passive partner, Robbie has conceived scenarios within which he is manipulated by machines, masturbated by them, and subjected to their wishes.

When he was nineteen, Robbie left home to attend college in another state. It was then that he had his first sadomasochistic experience. His partner was an older man who was active in the city's gay community. This experience was exciting and pleasurable, Robbie says. It involved only "light" S&M: exhibitionism, mild slapping, and slight humiliation. Robbie reports that he was so excited about this episode that he was laughing. He says that his partner was "amazed" by Robbie's reaction, since the man knew that Robbie was a novice in S&M. This is a common response on the part of "masters." They are continually astonished by how masochistic their slaves are, how much punishment they can take, and how deeply they are involved in the scenario. The fact that the masochist gets pleasure from the same act as he does is perpetually astounding to the sadist.

Despite having had masochistic fantasies involving women, Robbie has never had an opportunity to act on them. He did, however, become friends with a sadistic woman:

I met one S&M, sadistic-type woman in a bar in another city, but I never got into any S&M scenes with her because she said she could never do it to somebody she was friends with. . . . I got along fairly well with her. It was very nice, actually. She introduced me to some interesting people. Eventually, I got involved with other things and stopped seeing her.

Robbie's experience illustrates the findings of Andreas Spengler, who found that the opportunity for heterosexual men to make S&M contacts was severely limited. Bisexuals, on the other hand, had a much better chance for realizing their desires because they were willing to include other men as potential sex partners.

Robbie has a male friend with whom he regularly engages in sadomasochism. His friend, Robbie says, is a very good person and very affectionate. Although the other man can take both passive and aggressive parts, he is most often the master, since Robbie prefers to play slave.

Robbie enjoys being tied up (bondage) and whipped. The following portion of an interview with him nicely illustrates both his personal feelings about S&M and how the scene itself is a collaborative event, with the masochist having much of the control:

Interviewer: Do you go in for bondage?
Robbie: Um hum. Yes, I enjoy it very much.
I: Ropes, chains, or what?
R: Ropes, yeah. Could be anything.
I: Does he bind both your hands and feet?
R: That's the way it's done.
I: Do you get hung at all?
R: I think I got hung once or twice.
I: Do you use any kind of paraphernalia?
R: He has leather thongs that he uses for whips, and also this dog leash that makes a pretty good whip.
I: Do you mind getting whipped? Do you like it?
R: I like it. I find that pretty stimulating.
I: What kinds of things do you anticipate doing or working up to doing?

R: I like getting bound and whipped, because that's what most of my fantasies are.

I: Do you set a limit on that, like how hard he can whip you or where?

R: Not consciously. He wanted to put a specific number on it and I said, "No, go ahead and do what you want."

R: He enjoys that too?

R: I think he does.

I: Do you ever whip him?

R: Uh huh. Yeah. He likes to change roles.

I: How do you feel about that?

R: Fairly neutral about that. It doesn't do a lot for me.

Robbie is also a transvestite, but he does not dress up as a woman during S&M scenes. For those times, he wears a pair of bathing trunks that he has shortened. He first began cross-dressing when he was nineteen or twenty. He says that the desire to dress as a woman came upon him suddenly:

> One thing that did come suddenly was me becoming a transvestite. . . . This is something that's very clear in my mind. I started having dreams about transvestites for two nights in a row . . . and that gave me the idea I might enjoy it, so I tried it and I did.

Robbie was living back at home when he began to cross-dress. He found some old clothes in the attic. At first, he put them on surreptitiously. Later he began to be more open about his interest. He became involved in a gay organization and attended their dances and events dressed sometimes as a woman and at other times in "gender fuck" (i.e., dressing so as to strike a discordant note when viewed by "straight" people). He reports, for example, wearing a yellow chiffon dress and sporting a goatee at the same time. Robbie does not define himself as a "drag queen."[3] He says that he is a heterosexual transvestite. He reports getting sexual pleasure from dressing up in women's clothing.

Vito: An Identity in Transition

Vito is twenty-one years old and a sophomore in college. He has dark eyes and dark hair and is conventionally masculine in mannerisms and appearance. What is not conventional about Vito is his masochistic desires. They are further intertwined with both homosexual and heterosexual interests. During high school especially, Vito experienced a great deal of confusion and psychological pain over his sexual feelings:

> I was kind of mixed up for a while. Kind of like really mixed up. Because I didn't know whether I wanted to get into a relationship with a guy or a girl and I was really hung up on my masochism. . . . I really didn't know where I was at sexually.

In an attempt to figure things out, Vito read "psychology" books mostly and ordered books about homosexuality and masochism:

> I started reading a lot of books in late high school . . . just to discover things. Like, I ordered these books through the mail. All my books were basically on homosexuals or masochists, those kind of things. Even then, I guess, I was worried about it.

Vito comes from a lower middle-class Italian family. He was born in a large eastern metropolis and moved to the suburbs when he was eight years old. He has one sister, three years younger than him. He characterizes his mother as being "overprotective." Vito indicates some fear of his father and sees himself as not measuring up to some masculine ideal that the latter represented. This deep-felt sense of inferiority affected his relationship with girls during high school. Although he did date, Vito felt uncomfortable around them:

> I was always kind of uptight about dates in high school. . . . I probably just felt nervous because, I guess, coming from my background, which is Italian culture—and my father, when he was younger, was into boxing, and also my grandfather was a

construction worker—I think I always felt not manly enough. I always thought that if these girls really knew me, they wouldn't like me. I'm attracted to some girls, but I would like them to be the aggressor rather than me.

By the time he was about eleven years old, Vito had realized that he was attracted to males as well as to females. He did not act on this homosexual attraction, however, until he was much older. Vito recalls having had a crush on a best friend during high school, but he could never tell the other boy.

Vito had his first "petting" experience with a girl when he was thirteen. He met her at a party. She was the aggressor and allowed Vito to fondle her breasts. He felt very guilty about it afterward. Vito had a few other experiences with girls over the next few years, but they were limited to kissing and touching. He had not experienced sexual intercourse. At the age of eighteen, Vito decided to go to a prostitute:

> This was a different situation because, since I had gone out with a few girls and got really uptight with kissing and everything else, I figured that I should go to a prostitute and try something. . . . [It] was really a bad thing, because I didn't get off on it at all. And I think that after it, that's when I started saying, "You're definitely homosexual."

Vito began going to prostitutes to satisfy his masochistic desires. These scenes involved being verbally and physically humiliated and then masturbating. He did not have intercourse with these prostitutes. Vito says that he enjoyed these acts, but he did feel some guilt about them. It was also at about this time that Vito had his first homosexual experience. He met a young black man, in his mid-teens, with whom he established a sexual relationship. Unlike his previous relations with women, these homosexual experiences proved to be satisfying. "It was funny, when I got into it first, I might have been a little bit hung up about it. But then, that didn't last long, and I found the guy kind of attractive. So, I got into it."

At the age of nineteen, Vito had his first homosexual, sado-masochistic sexual experience. He had met a man at a meeting of an organization whose members included gay and heterosexual sadomasochists. Vito went home with the man and served as his slave. This initial exposure to gay S&M, however, proved to be disastrous for Vito. "With the prostitute I kind of liked it," Vito says, "but with this guy I didn't get into it at all."

Vito characterizes himself as "basically homosexual," but he is also interested in heterosexual relationships. He says that he is "fairly certain" about this. He stops short of considering himself bisexual, however, since he notes a greater attraction to men. Yet, he still finds himself attracted to women:

> It's funny. Most of the time I fantasize about guys; but there are times when I just look at a girl and fantasize about her. . . .I would definitely like to get into it if I could find the right woman.

Despite these fantasies, Vito is very wary of developing a heterosexual relationship. Some of his uncertainty lies in his feeling that he is not masculine enough. He is not an aggressive person and feels that this makes him unmanly. Encounters with females make him uncomfortable, because he feels that they expect him to be the aggressor:

> As of now, I'm still confused. . . . I don't know if I should go to a (gay) center and meet some guys or just meet some girl on campus. I really don't know. In a way, I'd rather meet up with some guy, because you don't have to worry about taking the initiative all the time or taking them out and buying them things. I'll see what happens, I guess. . . . Last semester, I definitely was interested in having a relationship with a few girls, but it just didn't work out.

Vito probably also recognizes that he has a greater probability of realizing his masochistic desires with men than with women. He did, in fact, note that the reason he went to prostitutes was that he assumed that women would reject him if he told them about his masochism.

Vito may have a long way to go in self-acceptance. He notes that he lacks self-confidence and that he feels insecure. He feels that his strong points include sincerity and being unprejudiced. Vito also has a lot of thinking to do about his sexual orientation. He has sought professional help in dealing with his feelings, but he does not believe that the psychologists whom he saw aided him very much. Given his ambivalence about women, it is quite probable that Vito will eventually become a participant in the gay S&M world, and limit his sexual activities to other men.

Conclusions

While the individual careers we have discussed are different in many ways there are, nevertheless, some common themes running through them. These similarities are all related to S&M as a form of social interaction. For example, the importance of learning both attitudes and techniques through a socialization process is evident in all of these careers. This is true even if an individual has had S&M fantasies from childhood as Daniel, Robbie, and Vito all report. Daniel relates that he first taught both Brenda and Jeanie how to dominate him, and then later he taught them how to be dominated. What he does not say, but what is implicit in his story, is that they, too, participated actively in the various scenarios and their responses taught him what did and did not work. Glen, Robbie, and Vito were all taught by persons who had previously been involved in S&M.

In order for an S&M scene to be successful, from the viewpoint of both partners, it must be collaboratively worked out. This is especially true for ongoing relationships like those reported by Daniel, Glen, and Robbie. Unless there is satisfaction on the part of both master (or mistress) and slave, the relationship will terminate. Thus, there must be agreement on the scene and consent given by both parties. Adjustments must be made by participants so that they are both stimulated. Vito's unhappy experience with a man is a case in point. In that situation only his partner was satisfied. Consequently, Vito was no longer willing to participate in S&M with this man. Robbie is fortunate in having a partner who can play both master and slave, since Robbie prefers the passive role. Yet, he also recognizes his friend's need to be dominated occasionally and, therefore, he will sometimes play master, even though, as he says, "It doesn't do a lot for me." Jeanie played the dominant role for Daniel for much the same reason.

Another finding apparent in all of these careers is that the S&M scene is a dynamic one with a constant feedback of "energy" between slave and master. This is most explicit when Daniel says of Brenda that, "her submission fed my dominance and vice versa." (Pat Califia notes the same sort of "energy flow" in her article in this volume.)

Finally, the importance of mutual love and affection for S&M couples is brought out by Daniel, Glen, and Robbie. They point out what sexologist Havelock Ellis noted long ago: that much sadomasochistic behavior is motivated by love.

Notes

1. We use the term "career" here in the way in which it has been defined by sociologist Erving Goffman: "Persons who have a particular stigma tend to have similar learning experiences regarding their plight, and similar changes in conception of self—a similar 'moral career' that is both cause and effect of commitment to a similar sequence of personal adjustments (*Stigma*, p. 32)."

2. "Punk" and "Wolf" are prison slang. A "wolf" is an aggressive, predatory man who takes the insertor role in anal sex, often as a rapist. He has a heterosexual self-identity. A "punk" is a weak, defenseless victim, often small and young, who takes the passive sexual role. He is sometimes homosexual in orientation.

3. A "drag queen" is a homosexual man who dresses in women's clothing. His wardrobe and mannerisms are often exaggerated. Drag does not usually have a sexual meaning. It is often done for fun and humor.

References

Califia, Pat. 1979. "A Secret Side of Lesbian Sexuality." *Advocate* (December 27): 19–23.

Ellis, Havelock. 1942. *Studies in the Psychology of Sex*, vol. 1, part 3. New York: Random House.

Goffman, Erving. 1963. *Stigma: Notes on the Management of Spoiled Identity*. Englewood Cliffs, N.J.: Prentice-Hall.

Spengler, Andreas. 1977. "Manifest Sadomasochism of Males: Results of an Empirical Study." *Archives of Sexual Behavior* 6: 441–56.

Charles Moser
and Eugene E. Levitt

An Exploratory-Descriptive Study of a Sadomasochistically Oriented Sample

The term *sadomasochism* (S/M) is usually construed to refer to an association between sexual arousal and physical and/or psychological pain (Haeberle 1978; Katchadourian and Lunde 1972/1975; Krafft-Ebing 1886/1965; McCary 1967/1973).[1] The physical pain is caused by behaviors which range from pinches, slaps, and bites to behaviors that may produce lesions or draw blood. The psychological pain encompasses feelings of helplessness, subservience, humiliation, and degradation. The psychological pain is brought about by verbal abuse, bondage, and "being forced" to do various acts. The range of behaviors and the paucity of previous research led us to decide on self-definition as an S/M participant as the least biased criterion for inclusion in the study.

Behaviors which appear to have some S/M characteristics occur in preliterate societies as well as among infra-human animals (Ford and Beach 1952; Kinsey, Pomeroy, Martin, and Gebhard 1953). They appear transhistorically in complex soci-

Reprinted from *The Journal of Sex Research* 23 (1987): 322–37. Copyright © 1987 by the Society for the Scientific Study of Sex. Reprinted by permission of the publisher and the author.

eties from ancient Egypt (Bloch 1935; Ellis 1903/1936) to the present, and in Indian (Kokkoka 1150/1965; Malla 1500/1964; Vatsyayana 450/1964), Oriental (Wedeck 1962), and Arab (Eulenberg 1934, cited in Ellis 1936) cultures. Unambiguous case examples of S/M have been reported in European literature since the late fifteenth century, and various S/M behaviors and fantasies are relatively common in contemporary civilizations (Hamilton 1929; Hariton 1972; Hunt 1974; Kinsey et al. 1953; Sue 1979).

General population surveys have not adequately established the proportion of the general population that identify S/M as part of their sexual pattern. Additionally, it is not clear if any specific behaviors can be classified as S/M unambiguously. Nevertheless, several studies suggest that S/M behavior in the United States is not rare and possibly common.

Hamilton (1929) interviewed 100 married men and 100 married women, fifty-five of whom were couples. He found 51% of the men and 32% of the women remember a time when they derived "pleasant thrills" from inflicting pain on either animals or humans, with 33% of the men and 19% of the women still reporting some trace of this tendency. He also found 28% of the men and 29% of the women remember a period of time when they derived "pleasant thrills" from pain being inflicted on them by other persons, with 20% of the men and 27% of the women still reporting some trace of this tendency.

Kinsey et al. (1953) found that 24% of the men and 12% of the women had at least some erotic response to sadomasochistic stories, and 50% of the men and 54% of the women had at least some erotic response to being bitten.

Hariton (1972) examined the fantasies during marital coitus of 141 married suburban women. She found that various submissive fantasies had incidences ranging from 19% to 49%, and these fantasies frequently recurred in 2% to 14% of the women, depending on the fantasy.

Stein (1974) studied (by surreptitious observation) men who patronized call girls. She observed 1,242 men with 64 call girls and categorized these men into nine types based on the apparent goal of the interaction. The "slave" category accounted for 13% of her sample. It is important to note that none of the call girls was a professional dominant, nor did they advertise this service.

Hunt (1974) did a questionnaire survey of sexual behavior involving 2,026 respondents in 26 cities. He found 4.8% of the men and 2.1% of the women had obtained sexual pleasure from inflicting pain, and 2.5 % of the men and 4.6% of the women had obtained sexual pleasure from receiving pain. Of these individuals, approximately 60% to 70% from each category reported obtaining sexual pleasure in that way in the last year.

Playboy (1976) contracted an independent research organization to survey 3,700 randomly selected college students from 20 colleges. They found 2% of the sample had tried and liked inflicting or receiving pain during sex and another 4% would like to try it. Another 3% of the sample had tried and liked bondage and/or master-slave role-playing. Of the total sample, approximately 12% of the women and 18% of the men indicated a willingness to try either or both of these behaviors. Also 5% of the men and 8% of the women reported sexual fantasies of infliction and/or receipt of pain.

Since the definition of S/M is not exact, speculation concerning the true incidence of S/M in the population is difficult. Nevertheless, using the lowest estimates and extrapolating from the studies reviewed above, it is clear that millions of people in the United States are involved in behaviors that most would classify as S/M. The large number of people involved and the paucity of research concerning the behavior suggests that further research is needed. The purpose of the present study is to describe a self-defined S/M sample: to ask who these people are, what do they do sexually, and how they feel about it.

There is a considerable body of clinical, theoretical, and speculative literature on sadomasochism (Levitt 1971; Moser 1979). However, there are few studies of S/M identified individuals. The only large-scale attempt of this type was carried out by Spengler (1975, 1977) in West Germany. Gosselin and Wilson (1980) did include a substantial number of sadomasochists (133 men and 25 women) in their sample, but they were primarily concerned with comparing various aspects of personality characteristics and the fantasy content of different groups of sexual variants.

Spengler (1977) studied 245 West German men by [a] questionnaire sent to advertisers in S/M contact magazines and to members of participating S/M clubs. Spengler's subjects were roughly evenly divided among individuals who self-defined as heterosexual, homosexual, or bisexual. He found that his respondents did not usually confide their S/M interests to family, friends, colleagues, or even their wives. The median frequency of sadomasochistic experiences was approximately five per year, with four to five different partners. Approximately 40% of the sample was involved in a relationship with a sadomasochistic partner for over a year. Spengler found that most of his sample had found a way to positive self-acceptance; the rate of attempted suicide is less than that of homosexual men in West Germany (Dannecker and Reiche 1974, cited in Spengler). Spengler found that most of his respondents alternated between the "passive" and "active" roles; exclusive role preference was rare. He found that 16% of his sample desired to have sex exclusively with S/M, with another 64% desiring sex predominately with S/M or equally with or without S/M. He further noted that 15% of his sample could attain orgasm only through sadomasochistic activity. Again, Spengler compared his sample to a sample of homosexuals (Dannecker and Reiche 1974) and found that masturbation frequency did not vary significantly. He did find that the highest masturbatory frequencies occurred among those who were most active with partners. He also found that the sadomasochistic "coming-out" occurred later than the average homosexual "coming out."

Our purpose was to investigate sadomasochism further by developing and studying a U.S. sample using a variation of Spengler's sampling tactics. Note that we collected data before Spengler's work was known to us. Although the similarity between questionnaires and sampling strategy are remarkable, it is not sound to compare results of two different surveys of different populations from different cultures statistically. Nevertheless, the similarity of the results is so striking that we believe that their comparison is worth further exploration.

Method

Respondents

The respondents were 178 men and 47 women, including 71 men and 23 women who attended a meeting of the Eulenspiegel Society in New York City and 18 men and 11 women who attended a meeting of the Society of Janus in San Francisco, both S/M support groups. Additionally, one man and six women found out about the study and requested to participate. These 90 men and 40 women all responded affirmatively to the question, "Do you define at least part of your sexuality as S/M?"

Another 88 men and 7 women completed a survey form printed in the *S/M Express,* an S/M-oriented magazine. These respondents were not asked the self-definition question, but the circulation of the magazine is so restricted that there is little chance that it would ever find its way into the hands of persons other than those with an S/M orientation.

Our male subsample turned out to be demographically similar to Spengler's (1977). We found a mean age of 38.2 years and a median age of 36, compared to Spengler's median in the 31–40 age bracket and approximate mean of 39 years. Both samples were better educated than the general population—70.2% of our sample were college graduates; another 24.7% had attended college. Spengler found 25% had completed college and another 15% had attended. The yearly income levels were also higher than the general population—33.3% of our subjects earned at least $25,000 per year and another 33.1% earned between $15,000 and $26,000— compared with 54% of Spengler's sample who earned over 1,500 Deutsche Marks per year, a comparable amount.

The mean age of the female subsample was 32.0, with 38.3%

having graduated from college and 44.7% having attended college. Only 8.8% of the female subsample earned more than $25,000, with another 13.3% earning between $15,000 and $25,000.

Approximately 95% of our sample was white. Although 43% of the men did not indicate a religious preference, 25% indicated they were Protestant, 15% Catholic, and 12% Jewish. Similarly, 62% of the women did not indicate a religious preference, with 11% Protestant, 11% Catholic, and 6% Jewish. Only 11% of the men and 9% of the women reported attending church as often as once a week, and 52% of the men and 62% of the women indicated that they never attended. Spengler (1977) did not report on either of these factors, but it may be assumed that his sample was largely Caucasian.

Instrument

The instrument[2] used was created specifically for this study. It contains 57 major items as multiple choice, one word fill-in, or checklist questions. These include demographics (eleven items), sexual identity or behavior (16 items), attitudes and responses to the S/M behavior (7 items), and the respondent's attitudes concerning S/M in general (4 items). There were 19 items that are not reported here, including one item which was ignored by most respondents and a psychological functioning inventory.[3] The survey form took between ten and thirty minutes to complete, with most respondents taking approximately fifteen minutes. The data were collected during the calendar year 1978.

Procedure

The *S/M Express* reprinted the survey in its December 1977 issue. *S/M Express* is a tabloid-type newsprint magazine containing explicit photographs, drawings, articles, stories, and advertisements which depict, by the magazine's own admission, sadomasochistic activities. The publisher of *S/M Express* claims a circulation of 20,000, so a response rate of 88 persons is approximately .5%. Although this appears quite small, no other study using a mail-in survey preprinted in an explicit magazine could be found to use in comparison. The editor of *S/M Express* included a short note which indicated that he knew the senior researcher, felt that it was a worthwhile study, and encouraged readers to complete and return the survey.

The surveys handed out at the meeting of S/M support groups were preceded by a short talk by the senior author in which it was indicated that the results would comprise his doctoral dissertation and that the purpose was to describe a self-defined S/M sample. At that time people were asked the self-definition question, "Do you define at least part of your sexuality as S/M?" Only those responding positively were included in the study. Some potential respondents asked about the meaning of the term S/M. It was explained only that S/M was another term for sadomasochism and that the potential subject's own definition was the important determinant. All the individuals at the Society of Janus meeting and approximately 85% of the individuals at the Eulenspiegel meeting completed the survey.

Results

Males

Subjects located themselves on each of two continua, based on how they thought of themselves rather than on behavior. The classical 7-point continuum of heterosexual-homosexual orientation (Kinsey, Pomeroy, and Martin 1948)[4] and an analogous 7-point continuum of dominance-submission were used. The present sample was largely heterosexual, with 84.8% indicating they were exclusively or predominantly heterosexual (Kinsey 0s, 1s, and 2s), whereas 12.9% indicated they were exclusively or predominantly homosexual (Kinsey 4s, 5s, and 6s). Only 2.2% of the sample responded that they were equally homosexual and heterosexual (Kinsey 3s), and a total of 7.8% of the sample indicated that they thought of themselves as having significant homosexual and heterosexual components (Kinsey 2s, 3s, and 4s).

The dominance-submission continuum (0 = *exclusively dominant*, 6 = *exclusively submissive*) was more evenly balanced between the dominance and submission poles. Of the sample, 43.6% indicated they were exclusively or predominantly dominant (0s, 1s, and 2s), and 42.5% were exclusively or predominantly submissive (4s, 5s, and 6s). There were 44.2% (2s, 3s, and 4s) of the sample that indicated that they had significant components of both dominance and submission in their self-definition. Only 8.6% indicated that they were exclusively dominant, and 7.5% indicated they were exclusively submissive. The indication is that our sample tended to be "switchable," interested in both dominant and submissive roles. (The term "switchable" is commonly used in the S/M support groups to define those interested in both dominant and submissive roles; other synonymous terms include "dual" and "middle.")

The expression "coming-out" has the same significance in the S/M milieu as among homosexuals. It denotes the entire process of recognizing the S/M inclination and adoption of an S/M-oriented identity. This psychosocial-ideational activity is distinguished from the first S/M experience, as it is for homosexuals. Both the first experience and the "coming-out" seem to be phenomena of adult life (Table 1). However, "coming-out" may also occur during adolescence: 26% of the sample reported a first S/M experience by age 16, and 10% indicated that they came out between the ages of 11 and 16.

On the average, first experience occurred at age 23 and "coming-out" at age 26 (Table 1). This difference is statistically significant. Nevertheless, first experience preceded coming-out for only 36% of the sample, and for 26% coming-out preceded first experience. For the remainder, the two circumstances occurred within the same year.

Also listed in Table 1 are some similar data collected by Spengler (1977). An estimated mean age at "first awareness" of

Table 1
The Onset of Sadomasochism

Age	West German* sample	Present sample	
	"First awareness"	"First experience"	"Coming out"
10 or younger	7%	12%	4%
11-12	10	4	6
14-16	25	10	4
17-19	15	9	12
20-24	20	22	20
25-29	12	22	22
30 and older	11	21	32
Estimated overall mean	20.3	22.9	25.9
N	237	178	178

Note. Chi-squares indicate that differences among all three categorizations ("first awareness," "first experience," and "coming out") are significant at the 1% level or beyond. The chi-square $(6, N = 415)$ for West German "awareness" versus the present study's "first experience" is 35.74, $p < .001$. The chi-square $(6, N = 415)$ for West German "awareness" versus the present study's "coming out" is 61.58, $p < .001$. The chi-square $(6, N = 356)$ for the present study's "first experience" versus the present study's "coming out" is 17.77, $p < .01$.

*West German data from Spengler (1977).

S/M tendency is approximately 20 years. Spengler's "first awareness" is not comparable to first experience in our sample nor is it the same as "coming-out." Regardless, age at first awareness in the Spengler sample is significantly earlier than either age at first experience or age at "coming-out" in our sample. These three criteria together may provide a more complete measure of the "coming out" process.

It was hoped that describing the respondents' behavior would yield information helpful in constructing a precise defini-

Table 2
Percentage of Total Sample Participating
in Various Sexual Behaviors

Behavior	Tried	Tried and Enjoyed*
Homosexual acts†	43.5	26.0
Group sex	40.1	29.4
Swinging (mate swapping)	22.0	17.5
Cross dressing	37.3	29.4
Fetish behavior	60.4	51.4
Incest	6.2	5.1
Bestiality	9.6	4.5
Burns	17.5	8.5
Humiliation	67.2	55.9
Branding	10.1	7.3
Tattoos	6.8	5.1
Enemas	42.3	29.9
Dildoes	56.5	48.0
Cock bindings	46.3	35.6
Leather	49.2	42.4
Mask	27.6	20.3
Piercing	14.7	11.3
Pins	18.1	13.6
Bondage	77.4	65.0
Boxing	6.2	5.1
Hot wax	37.3	24.3
Ice	41.3	26.6
Spanking	81.9	66.1
Whipping	65.0	49.7
Wrestling	28.2	22.0
Scat (coprophilia)	12.5	8.5
Water sports (urolangia)	44.6	33.3
Chains	52.6	40.7
Rubber	30.5	19.8
Hood	27.1	19.8
Biting	40.1	31.6
Face slapping	39.5	30.5
Kissing ass	58.2	48.0
Gag	49.2	36.2
Rope	64.9	54.2
Handcuffs	54.2	44.6
Blindfold	53.1	42.4

Table 2 (cont'd.)

Role Playing

Behavior	Tried	Tried and Enjoyed*
Teacher/student	32.2	25.4
Guardian/child	19.8	16.4
House servant	30.5	25.4
Master/slave (mental trip)	68.3	57.6
Master/slave (physical trip)	60.5	52.0
Master/slave (combination)	46.3	38.4

*Those who reported not enjoying the behavior might have either disliked the behavior or felt it was a neutral experience; we did not distinguish.

†Almost entirely oral-genital behaviors.

___

tion. We attempted to operationalize a definition of S/M by inquiring about participation in sexual behaviors falling into three categories: specific S/M behaviors, S/M role-playing behaviors, and sexual behaviors not specifically S/M. Percentages reporting having tried and enjoyed each behavior are shown in Table 2. The behaviors were listed on the survey form, with room to indicate behaviors not on the list. No new behaviors were reported.

Among the specific S/M behaviors, the most common were flagellation (spanking and whipping) and bondage (bondage, rope, chains, handcuffs, and gags). Such behaviors constitute the essence of the phenomenon known colloquially as "bondage and discipline." Percentages of the sample ranging from about half to more than 80% report having engaged in these S/M behaviors.

Some behaviors causing pain (ice, hot wax, biting, and face slapping), but relatively safe, are fairly common, reported by 37.3% to 41.3% of the sample. Another group of painful behaviors (burns, branding, tattoos, piercing, pins[5]), which are relatively more dangerous (i.e., more likely to cause medical problems), have been tried considerably less often, reported by 6.8% to 18.1% of the sample.

The term "humiliation" was deliberately left broad and unspecified. The high percentage of the sample reporting such behavior serves to illustrate that psychological pain is as much a part of S/M as physical pain. This is further illustrated by the data on S/M role-playing. These "scenes" are deliberately scripted fantasy activities in which one partner plays a role of a dominant person (teacher, guardian, master) relative to the other partner who plays the submissive role (student, child, slave). The relationship essence of the scene provides a context for the occurrence of various specific S/M behaviors such as whipping, spanking, bondage, humiliation, etc. A majority of our sample had engaged in some sort of master-slave scene. Teacher-student and guardian-child scenes are relatively less common.

A number of true-false belief and attitude statements were included in the survey to understand the S/M-identified individual better. A few members of the sample declined to respond; the percentages responding "true" to the statements in Table 3 are based on [numbers] ranging from 164 to 177.

About 95% of the sample found S/M activities as satisfying or more satisfying than "straight" sex, with 30% reporting that S/M activity was essential to a gratifying sexual experience. More than 85% believed that no one could guess their S/M inclinations from their day-to-day interactions, suggesting that the orientation is restricted to private, sexual behavior.

Between 5% and 6% of the sample seemed distressed by their involvement in S/M activities, as evidenced by their response to the statement, "I wish I were not into S/M." Another 5% to 6 % admitted to having been a patient in a psychiatric hospital, although not necessarily for reasons related to their S/M orientation. Approximately the same proportion of the sample felt that S/M is, in fact, a form of mental aberration, and more than 16% had consulted a professional person about their S/M inclinations.

Females

Spengler (1977) and Lee (1979) both had difficulty obtaining a female sample from an S/M population and concluded that few

Table 3
Beliefs and Attitudes:
Percentage of the Sample Endorsing Various Statements

	% endorsing
I wish I were not into S/M.	5.8
I have been a patient in a psychiatric hospital.	5.6
S/M may best be defined as a mental illness.	5.1
There have been times when I felt as though I was going to have a nervous breakdown.	32.2
I have sought help from a therapist regarding my S/M desires.	16.1
S/M sex is more satisfying than straight sex.	58.5
S/M sex is as satisfying as straight sex.	36.8
I need to be involved in an S/M scene to have a satisfactory sexual response.	30.2
There is a reasonable danger that S/M play will escalate to a truly dangerous extent.	29.9
From my day-to-day interactions, no one would guess my S/M orientation.	85.6
As a child, I remember getting erotic enjoyment out of being punished.	18.6

women are involved in the subculture if not the activity itself. Spengler believes that women involved in S/M activity do so only at the request of the male partner or for monetary reasons. Also, lesbian spokeswomen have stated, "S/M is a male perversion. There are no lesbians into S/M" (cited in Lee 1979, *Toronto Gaydays*, August 1978).

Despite these beliefs, we found evidence of a large number of women in the S/M subculture. The present study included 47 women, and several S/M organizations include substantial numbers of women. Califia (1979) reported that there are 200 members of a lesbian S/M club, SAMOIS, which published an anthology of lesbian S/M writings, *Coming to Power* (SAMOIS, 1981). There are S/M social groups which cater to either dominant men and submissive women or dominant women and sub-missive men. At social functions for these groups, members are usually required to attend with an opposite-sexed individual. Although there may be more men than women who desire to attend these functions, large numbers of women do attend. Fifty women would not be unusual at some events, and they are not the same fifty at each event. Therefore, we believe both that women are involved in the S/M subculture and are clearly involved in S/M activities. Additionally, Weinberg, Williams, and Moser (1984) did not have much difficulty finding women to interview for their study. Thus S/M is a sexual behavior like homosexuality where a significant percentage of women are practitioners, rather than a behavior like fetishism where women involved in the behavior are quite rare.

Our female subsample is not reported on in detail because of its small size and difficulty in comparing it to any other sample of women involved in variant sexual behavior. Nevertheless, these women tended to be more inclined to bisexuality than the men and to consider themselves more submissive than the men. They appear to be somewhat more experimental than the men, experiencing more different behaviors, both S/M and other sexual behaviors. The female subsample "came out" and engaged in their first S/M behavior at the same approximate ages as the males. The response to the 11 true-false items were essentially identical to the male subsample, except the women were more likely to feel as if they were having a nervous breakdown at times (60.0% to 32.2%), less likely to need S/M behavior to have a satisfactory sexual response (8.9% to 30.2%), and more likely to believe their interest in S/M could be guessed from their day-to-day interactions (34.1% to 14.4%).

Discussion

In any study on sexual behavior, the veracity of the responses must be questioned. Studies of behaviors with a negative stereotype (e.g., S/M) would be even more likely to include responses that are falsified in some way: The respondent might either try to shock the researcher or minimize the severity of the behavior. We cannot claim that the present study is totally devoid of such bias, but several factors suggest that any distortion is minimal. First, the senior author had worked in the S/M community for several years prior to data collection; thus he was well known to many of the respondents. The S/M organizations actively supported the research project both verbally and by providing time during their meetings for distribution and completion of the instrument. The instrument was reviewed by several people active in the S/M community to ensure that the wording would not be offensive and thus reduce negative reactions to the instrument. And lastly, several respondents indicated either verbally or in writing that they were pleased with the instrument and that they were happy that the project was undertaken. All these factors combined suggest that any intentional falsification was probably minor.

The respondents in both our sample and Spengler's (1977) sample were well-educated and affluent, suggesting the possibility that adoption of an S/M identity may somehow be related to these characteristics. Nevertheless, other explanations are more plausible. The sampling strategy could have skewed the sample. The better educated individuals (who are more likely to be affluent) may be more willing to participate in scientific research, more likely to join an S/M support group, or simply more likely to define their sexuality as S/M.

The data indicate that the polarities of S/M are less attractive to sadomasochists than variation between the two poles. Only 16.1% of our sample reported that they were exclusively either dominant or submissive, whereas more than 44.2% were markedly "switchable." Spengler's West German sample was more fixed in its preferences, though still quite "versatile," suggesting that efforts to study dominants compared to submissives may be futile.

Most of our respondents did not engage in an S/M activity,

nor realize this inclination, until a relatively late age. This might suggest that the inhibitions surrounding S/M are more durable and may take longer to break down. Another possible explanation is that in the developmental process, the realization of an S/M sexual preference usually occurs after determination of the individual's gender identity and sexual orientation.

Our subjects appeared to be interested in exploring different sexual behaviors and have attempted a wide range of both S/M and other sexual behaviors. For example, compared to general population estimates (Duckworth and Levitt 1985), substantially greater percentages of the present sample have engaged in, and enjoyed, group sex and swinging. The present sample also appeared to be more interested in variety than Spengler's German sample, though both samples seemed to be sexually adventurous. Our data do not enable us to determine if the sadomasochistic orientation itself is conducive to a broad range of sexual behaviors or if by violating one sexual taboo it becomes easier to break others.

Spengler (1977) also inquired about behaviors, but much more narrowly. Of the nine behaviors which are roughly comparable across samples, six occurred significantly more frequently in our sample than in Spengler's: pins (18% vs 6%), piercing (15% vs 6%), rubber (30% vs 12%), cross dressing (37% vs 14%), urolagnia (45% vs 10%), coprophilia (13% vs 5%). Those which did not differ were also the most common in both samples: whipping, bondage, and leather fetishism (see Table 2).

We found no single behavior that all S/M people found erotically stimulating, nor did we find that S/M was a *necessary* condition for a satisfying experience for most respondents. However, in the present sample, twice as many respondents required S/M activity to have a satisfactory sexual response compared to Spengler's (1977) sample (30.2% and 15%, respectively). From our data, sadomasochism appears to be a complex of behavioral phenomena that encompasses a wide variety of specific acts.

A preponderant majority of our subjects were well satisfied with their involvement in S/M activities. Not more than 6%

reported that they were emotionally disturbed about their involvement, although another 10%, approximately, reported that they had sought professional consultation about S/M inclinations. The difference in percentages suggests that those who sought professional help were seeking reassurance and permission, although our sampling technique may have excluded those who had negative feelings about the behavior.

It is surprising to find that distress, emotional illness, help-seeking, and negative belief are relatively unrelated to each other. Three of the six correlations are statistically significant, but the largest is only .28 (the correlation between expressing regret about being S/M inclined and the view that S/M is a mental illness). Evidently, the regretful respondents are not necessarily those who consider S/M to be an illness, nor those who have been hospitalized, nor those who had sought professional assistance.

About 30% of the sample believe that ordinary, gratifying S/M activities can escalate into an unscripted event that could cause serious harm. This view clashed with Lee's (1979) data, suggesting that the S/M subculture contains restraints that act to prevent such escalation. There are several possible explanations for this discrepancy. The most probable is that belief in the escalation hypothesis leads to the precautions that serve to prevent escalation. Belief may exist largely on a fantasy level, thereby lending a significant spice of excitement to the S/M scene without any true danger. Finally, Lee's sample was entirely homosexual; ours was largely heterosexual.

Despite some important intersample differences, the present data and West German data show considerable similarities. Both studies support the conclusions that S/M identified individuals: (a) tend to be relatively well educated and affluent; (b) tend not to identify themselves as exclusively dominant or submissive; (c) accept their interest in S/M relatively late in life; (d) engage in a variety of sexual behaviors, including those that are not S/M oriented; (e) engage in more extreme and dangerous S/M practices less often than other S/M practices; and (f) learn to accept themselves and their S/M identity without major reservations.

Notes

1. The problems of defining sadomasochism precisely are discussed by Moser (1979). They include the facts that: (a) the pain experience itself is altered during sexual arousal, (b) not all pain is arousing to avowed sadomasochists, and (c) some S/M experiences (e.g., restraint) are not painful.

2. Copies of the instrument can be obtained from the senior author.

3. The same psychological functioning inventory used by Weinberg and Williams (1975) was implanted in the present instrument. The results indicated that S/M-identified individuals functioned as well as Weinberg and Williams' sample and the control group. Problems with comparing slightly different versions of the inventory, size of the sample, and inability to match subjects on all demographic criteria make statistical analysis inappropriate.

4. In the Kinsey scale 0 is exclusively heterosexual, 6 is exclusively homosexual, and 3 is equally homosexual and heterosexual.

5. The correlation between pins and piercing is .97; between burns and branding, .93. These coefficients indicate that the correlated behaviors were very probably interpreted as synonymous by most of the respondents.

References

Bloch, I. 1935. *Strangest Sex Acts*. New York: Falstaff Press.

Califia, P. 1979. "A Secret Side of Lesbian Sexuality." *The Advocate* (December 27): 19–23.

Dannecker, M., and R. Reiche. 1974. *Der gewohnliche Homosexuelle*. Frankfurt: Fischer.

Duckworth, J., and E. E. Levitt. 1985. "Personality Analysis of a Swinger Club." *Lifestyles: A Journal of Changing Patterns* 8: 35–45.

Ellis, H. 1936. *Studies in the Psychology of Sex*. New York: Random House. (Original work published 1903)

Eulenberg, A. 1934. *Algolagnia*, trans. H. Kent. New York: New Era Press.

Ford, C. S., and F. A. Beach. 1952. *Patterns of Sexual Behavior*. New York: Harper.

Gosselin, C., and G. Wilson. 1980. *Sexual Variations: Fetishism, Sadomasochism and Transvestism*. New York: Simon and Schuster.

Haeberle, E. 1978. *The Sex Atlas*. New York: Seabury Press.

Hamilton, G. V. 1929. *A Research in Marriage*. New York: Boni.

Hariton, E. 1972. *Women's Fantasies during Sexual Intercourse with Their Husbands: A Normative Study with Tests of Personality and Theoretical Models*. Ph.D. diss., City University of New York (University Microfilms No. 73–2839).

Hunt, M. 1974. *Sexual Behavior in the 1970s*. Chicago: Playboy Press.

Katchadourian, H., and D. Lunde. 1975. *Fundamentals of Human Sexuality*, 2d ed. New York: Holt, Rinehart and Winston. (Original work published 1972)

Kinsey, A. C., W. B. Pomeroy, and C. E. Martin. 1948. *Sexual Behavior in the Human Male*. Philadelphia: Saunders.

Kinsey, A. C., W. B. Pomeroy, C. E. Martin, and P. H. Gebhard. 1953. *Sexual Behavior in the Human Female*. Philadelphia: Saunders.

Kokkoka. 1965. *The Hoka Shastra*, trans. A. Comfort. New York: Stein and Day. (Original work published ca. 1150 A.D.)

Krafft-Ebing, R. von. 1965. *Psychopathia Sexualis*, trans. F. S. Klaf. New York: Bell. (Original work published 1886)

Lee, J. 1979. "The Social Organization of Sexual Risk." *Alternative Lifestyles* 2: 69–100.

Levitt, E. E. (1971). "Sadomasochism." *Sexual Behavior* 1 (6): 68–80.

Malla, K. 1964. *The Anganga Ranga*, trans. F. Arbuthnot and R. Burton. New York: Lancer Books. (Original work published ca. 1500 A.D.)

McCary, J. 1973. *Human Sexuality*, 2d ed. New York: Van Nostrand Reinhold. (Original work published 1967)

Moser, C. A. 1979. *An exploratory-descriptive study of a self-defined S/M (sadomasochistic) sample*. Ph.D. diss., Institute for Advanced Study of Human Sexuality, San Francisco, Calif.

Playboy, eds. 1976. "What's Really Happening on Campus." *Playboy* (October), pp. 128–31, 160–64, 169.

SAMOIS, eds. 1981. *Coming to Power*. Palo Alto, Calif.: Up Press.

Spengler, A. 1975. *Sadomasochists and their subculture: Results of an empirical study*. Paper presented at the annual meeting of the International Academy of Sex Research, Hamburg, Germany (August).

———. 1977. "Manifest Sadomasochism of Males: Results of an Empirical Study." *Archives of Sexual Behavior* 6: 441–56.

Stein, M. 1975. *Lovers, Friends, and Slaves*. New York: Berkeley Publishing.

Sue, D. (1979). "Erotic Fantasies of College Students During Coitus." *The Journal of Sex Research* 15: 299–305.

Vatsyayana. 1964. *Kama Sutra.* New York: Lancer Books. (Original work published ca. 450 A.D.)

Wedeck, H. 1962. *Dictionary of Aphrodisiacs.* London: Peter Owen.

Weinberg, M., and C. Williams. 1975. *Male Homosexuals.* New York: Penguin Books.

Weinberg, M., C. Williams, and C. Moser. 1984. "The Social Constituents of Sadomasochism." *Social Problems* 31: 379–89.

SCENES
S&M INTERACTIONS

Introduction

This section opens with Thomas S. Weinberg's article, "Sadism and Masochism: Sociological Perspectives." Weinberg discusses some of the subcultural aspects of the heterosexual S&M world. This selection represents a preliminary attempt to view sado-masochism as a theoretically approachable phenomenon, drawing upon frame analysis to bring out the germane features of the S&M scene. Frame analysis, developed by sociologist Erving Goffman, conceives of human interaction as being bounded or "framed" by social definitions that give the behavior a specific contextual meaning. The meaning of what is happening is shared, and a variety of "keys" are used to cue participants into what is "really going on." Frames not only define interaction, but they also control and restrict it as well. They set forth mutually agreed upon limits, which participants accept as inviolable. So, for example, what may appear to the uninitiated observer as a violent act may really be a theatrical and carefully controlled "performance" from the perspective of the participants. Thus, we find in this article what is perhaps the first attempt to frame S&M in the dramaturgical mode, a conceptualization originally alluded to by Gebhard.

Pat Califia's essay, "A Secret Side of Lesbian Sexuality," is valuable in a number of ways. Like the Kamel "Leather Career" and "Leathersex" articles elsewhere in this collection, she focuses on a specific S&M subculture. In her discussion of the lesbian sadomasochistic world, Califia gives us an insider's first-hand account both of S&M interaction and of how a participant (in this case Califia herself) structures, defines, and feels about what is going on. In this sense, her article links both identities and scenes by illustrating how "frames" are constructed in the S&M world to serve the needs of individual S&Mers.

The ethnographic research of both James Myers and Joel I. Brodsky provides insight into two specific subworlds of the S&M community. Myers studied nonmainstream body modification (e.g., genital piercing, branding, burning, and cutting) through participant observation and interviews. Although earlier researchers found that nonmainstream body modification was not a very common practice (e.g., Moser and Levitt 1987 found that just 17.5 percent of their sample had participated in burning, 10.1 percent had been tattooed, and 14.7 percent had been pierced; Spengler 1977 reported that 7 percent of his subjects had employed glowing objects and 4 percent had used knives and razor blades), Myers notes that such permanent body alterations are becoming increasingly popular. He presents several possible motivations for involvement in nonmainstream body modification, including those of participating in a rite of passage, as a means of affiliating oneself with a desired group, and as a test of trust and loyalty. He thus adds to the development of a *sociological* theory of S&M subcultures.

Another important contribution of the Myers study is that his research provides us with qualitative information on women in the S&M scene. It thus importantly supplements the work of Moser and Levitt, and Breslow and his colleagues, which also appear in this volume.

Brodsky (1993) provides a retrospective ethnography of the Mineshaft, a gay male leather bar which existed in New York City until 1985, when it was closed down by state authorities. By describing interaction within the setting from the viewpoint of a participant, he answers the question, "What did going to the Mineshaft do for those who went there?" (p. 234). His answer is that it served to organize risk reduction, providing a safe place in which S&M experimentation could occur in the presence of experienced S&M practitioners. It was a setting that facilitated socialization into the leathersex subculture, serving as a "focal point for symbolic ritual activity among gay men" (p. 239). Similar to Myers, Brodsky notes the importance of rites of passage and symbols of affiliation for participants in the S&M world.

Thomas S. Weinberg

Sadism and Masochism: Sociological Perspectives

Sadism and masochism are two varieties of sexual behavior of which description and analysis have been largely lacking in the professional literature. Sadomasochism has generally been described only by psychiatrists; consequently, the social aspects of this behavior have been almost completely ignored. Sadomasochism has been of interest to the legal profession and the lay public only when some highly publicized crime with sadomasochistic overtones has occurred. Examples of these instances include the infamous English "Moors" murders (*Newsweek*, May 2, 1966), the sexual mutilation and killing of William Velten in New Mexico in 1974 (Footlick and Smith 1975), and the so-called "trash bag murders" which were recently uncovered in California (*Buffalo Courier-Express*, July 4, 1977). Sociologists of deviance have largely neglected sadomasochistic (S&M) behavior. Some . . .basic texts in the sociology of sexual behavior do devote a few paragraphs or pages to this behavior (DeLora and

Reprinted from: *The Bulletin of the American Academy of Psychiatry and the Law*, vol. 6, no. 3 (1978): 284–95. Reprinted by permission of the author.

119

Warren 1977; Gagnon 1977; Pengelley 1978), but their observations are neither systematic nor theoretical. A paper (by Weinberg and Falk [1978]) attempts a more systematic overview of the S&M subculture, but it lacks any theoretical organization. Journalists (Coburn 1977; Halpern 1977) have also examined the sadomasochistic subculture, but their work, too, is largely descriptive and usually confined to reporting events at an S&M organization such as the Till Eulenspiegel Society in New York City.

Although attempts to theoretically organize and explain sadomasochism as a social phenomenon have not been made by sociologists, sociological literature and theory do provide a number of helpful starting points. There is, for example, a large literature on subcultural deviance which might be explored. Frame analysis, role theory, interactionist, phenomenological, and ethnomethodological perspectives might be profitably used to gain some insight into the world of sadists and masochists. This paper represents a tentative attempt to apply some of the current theoretical perspectives in sociology to a study of the social organization of consensual sexual violence.

[My] data include fully transcribed interviews with participants in the S&M scene, including "amateurs" and professional "dominatrixes," materials from S&M magazines, literature and flyers from sadomasochistic organizations, and so forth. The S&M world includes professional and nonprofessional segments and both "straight" and "gay" subworlds (*Time*, September 8, 1975). Members of this world, however, may not necessarily perceive themselves along these lines. There are blendings and blurrings and crossings over from one part of this world to another. Advertisers in S&M contact publications often make a point of their "flexibility," "versatility," or "bisexuality."

There are two central features of the sadomasochistic world. The first is that much of this behavior occurs within a subcultural context. This is not surprising, since by its very nature, participation in this behavior requires at least two individuals, and necessitates some degree of social organization in order to be consummated. It is, of course, not uncommon for individuals to engage in solitary autoerotic sadomasochism, sometimes with tragic results (Dietz 1978). A second feature of the sadomasochistic world is that this social organization is "framed" (Goffman 1974) in terms of fantasy, as a kind of theatrical production. Fantasy and theatricality are reflected, for example, in the roles available to players, their relations to one another, the kinds of scenes that are enacted, and the argot of the group.

The S&M Subculture

Deviant subcultures form, according to Albert K. Cohen (1955), when individuals with common problems of adjustment come into communicative interaction with one another. The subculture, as a system of beliefs and values generated through this interaction, serves to help the individuals solve these problems. Although Cohen's work was concerned with delinquent youths, his ideas are applicable to other sorts of subcultures. People with sadomasochistic interests, like individuals with other nonmodal desires such as gays (Weinberg 1976), often recognize these needs quite early but are unable to act upon them, for they do not know that a world of their "own" (Goffman 1963) exists. They often feel isolated and "sick." Often their exposure to other sadists and masochists is fortuitous, as illustrated in the following conversation between an interviewer (I) and a respondent (R):

I: Okay, you were going to talk a little about S&M.
R: Yeah, I'm not really sure where to start. I've found I really enjoyed it and always had fantasies about it. It's really good. What are some of the things you'd like to know about?
I: Well, for example, how did you first start thinking that you were interested in S&M and how did you eventually act out on it and so on?
R: Okay. Well, my fantasies, ever since early childhood, have always been masochistic. . . . And then, when I was devel-

oping a gay identity, my fantasies changed only a little. And I never really acted upon it, until I came onto somebody in (city) who was a sadist. And he was really an interesting person. He opened up a very fancy restaurant. . . . There's a gay community council in (city), and they held some of their meetings over in his restaurant. And I decided that I wanted to attend one . . . and also the restaurant manager was there and we just got to talking, you know. . . . And after everybody left, he just started talking to me and he just kind of closed off a part of the restaurant, and we just started having sex there and then we went into his office and more over there and then we went down to his room where he seemed to store dishes and stuff, it was completely closed off, and it got real heavy in there. And he treated me really special, I thought, giving me free food after that and giving me a ride home with somebody else. But after that I didn't see him because some of his friends seemed to have nicknames like "Godfather" and so forth.

I: Did you get into an S&M scene with him then?

R: Right.

I: What did you do? Did he tie you up? Did he initiate it or did you or what?

R: He did.

I: What did he do?

R: He didn't have any equipment or anything. There was a lot of slapping and he wanted me to masturbate in front of him and he wanted me to talk to his cock.

I: And then what happened? You said you didn't see him again?

R: Right. Afterwards, I really felt kind of elated and kind of like laughing and he said, "You're amazing!" Like he was completely flabbergasted by it.

I: Why, because you enjoyed it?

R: Yeah. I think that was it.

Other respondents met people interested in S&M through already established sadomasochistic organizations:

I: Can you tell me about (your first sadomasochistic act) and how it happened and so on?

R: Well, there's this place in New York called the Eulenspiegel Society. I don't know whether you ever heard of it; it's kind of a place where all people, they call it sexual minority people, go, people with sadomasochistic behavior or gay people go there, straight people, bisexuals, some transvestites, a kind of real liberal place. And I met this guy there and he said he was interested in getting together in this act, this sadomasochistic thing. And I said, "Yeah, I'd like to try it." And, we went to his house, apartment in New York and I've always had fantasies around that area . . . but with this guy, I didn't get into it at all. I mean, you know, the fact of being tied up and getting hit with a belt. I just, I don't know, I thought I could get into it, but once it happened I just didn't get into it at all. I didn't like being fucked up the ass either. It hurt me.

I: Did you reciprocate? Did you do it to him?

R: No.

Some people discover the S&M world through other, related, deviant worlds. A professional dominatrix, for example, told the researcher that she had learned about sadomasochism through contacts with customers in a brothel:

I: How did you decide that you were going to specialize in S&M?

R: Well, I decided that because when I went into the houses to work I saw that that entailed more money. And it was interesting to me. Like, the first time I ever did it, like I took over the house and I was shooting so much drug, I was spending so much money on drug, I would be up one minute and I'd be back down on the streets the next minute. Then I'd fall into something else. And I was working in this house. The house was a very good house. This is how I first found out about *Screw* magazine and one day a guy came in and he needed somebody to do a dominance session with him. And I didn't know what to do. And one of the girls just said to me, "Well, here's some material," and told me what to do and I went up there and I took it from there and it was just something that came naturally to me.

I: What did he want you to do, do you remember?

R: It was a bondage session and a verbal humiliation session with whips.

I: What do you do during verbal humiliation sessions?

R: Well, you know, some guys just don't like anything else except to be verbally humiliated. You tell them that they're disgusting, you know, "You dirty son of a bitch." And, "You're this. And you're a pervert and look how ugly you are." All kinds of the worst things that you can think about somebody just to verbally humiliate them. You know, like maybe stand on their heads. Or stand on them and you're talking to them and just make them feel as low as you can. You know, having them on the ground. Just stepping on somebody's head like that. People pay for it.

The other side of the professional S&M scene is reported by a man whose first sadomasochistic acts were with a prostitute:

R: This is a hangup (I had) with girls, because what I really was into was kind of a sadomasochistic thing, you know, and when I was young I really felt I could never talk to any girls about that. But then when I tried a few sexual acts with prostitutes and that, in that way, it was kind of enjoyable although there was no intercourse because it was more money. And so it was just kind of a scene with just masturbation.

I:　And how did you feel about these experiences?

R:　I really enjoyed them, but I felt guilty about it. Deep inside there was a lot of guilt. But I really enjoyed it.

I:　Why did you go to the prostitutes, then?

R:　Why?

I:　Yeah.

R:　I don't know. I guess just because I figured that a girl wouldn't. I don't know, a regular girl would be kind of turned off by, you know, fantasy called "abnormal" or "deviant."

Novices in sadomasochism may also attempt to make contacts through S&M magazines, sometimes advertising themselves as beginners, "New and into bondage," "New to these adventures but not turned off," and so forth.

Once subcultures are formed, they provide their members with techniques for engaging in certain kinds of behavior and with ideologies, "motives, drives, rationalizations, and attitudes" (Sutherland and Cressey 1960) that serve to normalize and even to elevate the individual's needs and behavior. In the case of S&M, techniques are taught not only through personal contact, but through letters and stories appearing in sadomasochistic publications. Some advertisers in contact magazines, in fact, offer to "train" and "dominate" respondents by mail. Numerous companies produce and advertise an endless variety of devices, costumes, and paraphernalia used in the "training" of S&M devotees.

The development of apologias, attitudes, and ideologies supportive of S&M appears to be more important than the dissemination of specific techniques for restraining people and inducing pain and discomfort. Statements of sadomasochistic organizations serve to justify and celebrate the activities of their members. For example, a Eulenspiegel flyer says:

What *is* S&M? Does the phrase conjure up vague visions of DeSade or Torquemada, or perhaps at best *The Story of O*? The subject has always been cloaked in fear and speculation, largely because of the shroud of ignorance born of traditional sex taboos.

The *Eulenspiegel Society* is an organization devoted to shedding light and joy on this neglected area of sexual fulfillment. Eulenspiegel is not in any sense a sex club or swingers' organization, but a discussion and consciousness-raising group that explores the cultural and psychological nature of *sexual dominance and submission*, sadism and masochism. It is the aim of this organization to promote better understanding and self-awareness of these drives so that they may be enjoyed as a part of a full sex life, rather than set aside out of fear or guilt.

Malibu Publications, which publishes the magazine *Amazon*, displays a similar rationale for sadomasochistic behavior in a flyer advertising their magazine:

As the name indicates this is a contact magazine devoted exclusively to devotees of S&M/B&D.[1] It was launched just over a year ago in context with the philosophy that inasmuch as every human being harbors masochistic and/or sadistic tendencies, why not bring S&M/B&D out of the "closet" by tastefully presenting the subject as the normal sexual indulgence it really is. *Amazon* has achieved this! It provides the average person with a publication that reveals S&M/B&D as a normal form of sexual activity and alleviates any feelings of guilt and/or perversion arising from long held misconceptions.

These statements fall into the general category of what have been called "accounts," "linguistic device(s) employed whenever an action is subjected to valuative inquiry" (Scott and Lyman 1968). More specifically, accounts are statements "made by a social actor to explain unanticipated or untoward behavior. . . . An account is not called for when people engage in routine, common-sense behavior in a cultural environment that recognizes that behavior as such" (Scott and Lyman 1968). The kinds of accounts presented here are illustrative of what Scott and Lyman call "justifications." "Justifications are accounts in which one accepts responsibility for the act in question, but denies the pejorative quality associated with it" (Scott and Lyman 1968). In particular, one type of justification explicitly used in these apologias is a device that Scott and Lyman (1968) term "self-fulfillment." That is, the writers of these statements do not simply normalize sadomasochistic behavior for the initiated; instead, they attempt to enlighten outsiders about the "joys" of this behavior. Thus, the importance of these accounts is that they are not merely concocted by individual, isolated actors. They are, instead, socially produced, taught, reinforced, and continually reaffirmed by members of a given subculture or group. The group thereby does for the individual what he cannot do for himself. It provides him with external justifications for his desires and behavior. In a word, the subculture normalizes his orientation for him. Some of these accounts, more accurately, are "techniques of neutralization," similar in function and often in tone to those produced by gangs of delinquent youths (Sykes and Matza 1957).

These sorts of apologias represent what Abraham Kaplan has called "reconstructed logic," in contrast with what he terms "logic-in-use" (Kaplan 1964). Reconstructed logic is an *ex post facto* idealization rather than an accurate description of participants' motives as ongoingly displayed in actual S&M situations (logic-in-use). Compare, for example, the Eulenspiegel statement with journalistic descriptions of actual Eulenspiegel meetings and events (Coburn 1977; Halpern 1977) or, for instance, with the statement of one participant, a professional dominatrix:

> Well, eventually I just, they were just business to me. I really didn't care for them at all. They were just money. It was just like getting in there and getting out of there. It was just a business, that's all. I hated them, especially when I got into the S&M thing, you know. Then I took out all my frustrations on them. I was very brutal.

Fantasy and the Theatrical Frame

It is impossible to attempt to develop an understanding of the sadomasochistic subculture without examining the place of fantasy and theatricality in this world. The S&M scene is a fantasy world and can be most effectively understood in that light. Here we can profitably draw from the insights of Erving Goffman, especially with reference to his work on frame analysis (Goffman 1974). Frameworks, according to Goffman, are perspectives or "schemata of interpretation," which, when applied by an individual to events, render "what would otherwise be a meaningless aspect of the scene into something that is meaningful . . . each primary framework allows its user to locate, perceive, identify, and label a seemingly infinite number of concrete occurrences defined in its terms" (Goffman 1974, p. 21). The kinds of frameworks with which we are concerned here are social frameworks. The theater is an example of one sort of social frame. Goffman notes that the primary frameworks of a particular social group are a central element of its culture (Goffman 1974). These frameworks are embedded within the language of the group (Goffman 1974). The language itself provides rules for their application within specific contexts, as well as defining particular roles, identities, and relationships within these contexts. The special argot of S&M works in this way.

Related to Goffman's discussion of frameworks is his concept of "keys" and "keying." A "key," according to Goffman is "the set of conventions by which a given activity, one already meaningful in terms of some primary framework, is transformed into something patterned on this activity but seen by the participants to be something quite else. The process of transcription can be called keying" (Goffman 1974, pp. 43–44). An example of keying would be action that appears to be fighting but has been transformed into play by the "combatants." Participants in the activity are consciously aware of the systematic alteration that is going on.

S&M activity appears to fall within what Goffman calls the "theatrical frame." Within this frame, various sorts of keyings are used by the participants: those which transform what might appear to an outsider to be violence into make-believe or a kind of play-like behavior, those which set limits, those which affect role switchings and the dominance order, and so on. An important aspect of any dramatic scripting, such as those which occur during a sadomasochistic episode, is that unlike the situation in the real, everyday world where a certain degree of uncertainty obtains, participants in this activity have the opportunity to " 'play the world backwards,' that is, to arrange now for some things to work out later that ordinarily would be out of anyone's control and a matter of fate or chance." "In the case of make-believe," as Goffman puts it, "the individual can arrange to script what is to come, unwinding his own reel" (Goffman 1974, p. 133). This is exactly what occurs in the S&M world. Participants interact within a particular (theatrical) frame, collaboratively setting specific limits to the scene. This limit setting is critical, as a respondent indicates:

> Usually, sometimes, when you have a new client, what I used to do was I used to sit down and I would talk to them first and find out exactly what they wanted. Because sometimes you can get into a session with somebody and get very brutal and that's not what they want. There's heavy dominance and there's light dominance and there's play acting, roles, all different kinds. So the best thing to do is to sit down and talk to somebody first, initially.

Devotees of S&M frequently indicate that it is the masochist who controls the interaction in a sadomasochistic episode. That is, he sets the limits by keying this activity as make-believe, something which is to be understood as not the "real thing." A male masochist, who defines himself as "bisexual," explains how he works out limits with his partner:

I: Someone tells me that in an S&M situation it's really the masochist who has all the control.

R: Uh huh.

I: Is that true?

R: Could be. I just read in (publication) that there's maybe no such difference as between passive and aggressive partners. That you can never be entirely passive or aggressive. . . . And, if I didn't want him to do something, I'd let him know. And he'd have to stop right there, because there's also, like, limits.

I: Is there a kind of understanding between S&M people, that you set out limits? You set these limits out before, or . . . ?

R: Before. Before each act. He liked to press me to do heavier and heavier things. But, uh, you definitely have to have a limit, before you go further. So, if I don't like it, you're not going to go on.

I: Are there certain things that you don't do?

R: Um huh. Yes.

I: Like what?

R: I really don't like being pissed on. Even though there's actually no pain involved. And, he wanted to stick pins in me. But he just gets near me with a pin and I jump ten feet.

An interesting phenomenon in the sadomasochistic world is what appears to be an overrepresentation of "dominant" women and "submissive" men. In a content analysis of two issues each of *Latent Image* and *Amazon*, popular S&M contact publications, the preferences (either "dominant" or "aggressive," or "submissive" or "passive") of advertisers who indicated an orientation were distributed as shown in Table 1.

In the large proportion of cases, "submissive" women sought other women or couples. This was also true for couples in which the woman was the submissive partner. Some of the submissive women who advertised appear to really be half of a couple. In any event, it does not seem to be the case that "submissive" women seek out dominant men. As a recent text in "sex and human life" observes, "it is commonly the case that sadistic men cannot find a masochistic female partner" (Pengelley 1978, p. 154).

The presence of high proportions of dominant women and submissive men in a society in which men are supposed to be aggressive and women are defined as passive presents an inter-

Table 1
Self-Characterizations as "Dominant" or "Submissive" by
Advertisers in S&M Contact Magazines

Magazine, Issue	Males N=201		Females N=480			Couples N=93		
	Dominant	Submissive	Dominant	Submissive	Both Dominant	Female Dominant/ Male Submissive	Male Dominant/ Female Submissive	Both Submissive
Latent Image, No. 11	8	27	39	5	2	9	6	2
Latent Image, No. 12	16	14	46	3	3	3	9	2
Amazon, No. 4	24	45	105	28	8	1	6	3
Amazon, No. 6	23	44	207	47	16	5	13	5
TOTAL	71	130	397	83	29	18	34	12

esting paradox which may be resolved by referring to the theatrical frame. Goffman observes that "frequent role switching occurs during play, resulting in a mixing up of the dominance order found among the players during occasions of literal activity" (Goffman 1974). Within a fantasy scene, traditional sex roles may be reversed without threatening the participants, if it is defined as "just make-believe." Roles are reversed, however, only in the sense that an individual who is "really" an adult male finds himself subservient to another who is "really" a female. But since the interactants are frequently acting out roles different from the ones which they "normally" occupy, very often the dominance order of the "real world" is sustained. That is, in the "real" world, some people (e.g., adults) have rights over others (e.g., children) where such rights include the administration of certain forms of corporal punishment, violence, and the like. Traditionally, males have such rights over females, hence, women's complaints at being "treated like children," and so forth. In a recent paper, for example, West and Zimmerman (1977) find that there are "striking similarities between the pattern of interruptions in male-female interchanges and those observed in the adult-child transactions" and interpret this to mean that "females have an analogous status to children in certain conversational situations (which) implies that the female has restricted rights to speak and may be ignored or interrupted at will"(West and Zimmerman 1977, p. 525).

Much S&M activity follows general social-organizational patternings, so that when the relations are "reversed" (e.g., when the man gets beaten, degraded, etc.) metaphors like "governess"/"child," "mistress"/"slave," "teacher"/"pupil," and so forth are used to invoke a conventional patterning anyway. A dominatrix, when asked why she thought men had developed their particular interests, answered in terms of their childhood backgrounds, and pointed out that they often took child-like roles within the S&M interaction:

I: Have you ever tried to figure out why some of these people are into some of the things they're into?

R: Well, I didn't have to figure it out. I've asked them. A lot of them have talked to me about it. A lot of it stems from the way their mothers were, experiences they've had in childhood. A lot of it stems from, you know, things that have happened to them when they were kids. Something that impressed them when they were a child and it stayed with them for the rest of their lives. I had one guy that, I guess, his mother was on his back all the time. Another guy used to watch the spankings, and another guy that used to come in and I used to have to play his big sister and I'd stand in the bathroom while he would take something of mine, pretending that he was taking it out of the drawer and I'd have to come in and say to him, "What are you doing?" you know, and we'd go through the whole act. . . . I used to have a guy that used to come in, he used to like to put on diapers and play like you're a baby and you're supposed to pee on yourself or in a diaper, and things like that.

Some males who take the submissive role do so only when they are dressed as women. Others pretend to be dogs, horses, or other animals. S&M contact magazines are filled with ads from male transvestites and others who wish to participate in sadomasochistic activities in roles other than that of adult male, and from women who sustain these kinds of fantasies:

GODDESS ADRENA COMMANDS all humble & obedient servants to beg for application into her male DOG TRAIN-ING classes. Beg to be my lap dog douche bag mouth & crawl beneath me always!

All bad boys int. in spanking, B&D, S&M, female domina-tion, or enemas write to Queen Linda, Glendale.

Well trained Dominant and exotic TV arranging for "Dude" ranch with fully equipped stables, dungeon, leather gar-ments, etc. All dominant fems invited to participate. Male "Studs" must qualify through series of private training ses-sions. For further details & photos, write. San Francisco.

White male, 30, Bi-sexual, wishes to meet attractive, domi-nant woman or T.V. Couples OK if she is dominant. Dress me in frilly, silky, women's things and I will be your FR. maid or sisterly companion. Also enjoy leather & rubber. Lasting relationship possible. No professionals. Send photo and phone. Can & will travel, particularly to the N.E.

Men who are submissive would appear to be able to recon-cile these needs with the societal pressures on males to be active, dominant, and superordinate to women by donning a special role within an S&M episode. Thus, it is the actor as a "child" ("slave," "female maid," "dog," etc.) who is being beaten, de-graded, humiliated, and so forth, and not the person in his "actual social identity" (Goffman 1963) as an adult male. By tak-ing a role which is not "really" his "own," the individual reinforces the definition of the situation as "play," "make-believe," "fantasy," and the like. This enables him to segregate the S&M situation from his everyday life. Professional prostitutes and dominatrixes often point out the apparent ease and rapidity with which clients can slip in and out of these roles (von Cleef 1971). A good deal of this has to do with keying of the activity. Specialized argot and terminology serves to cue the activity in and out for the participant. Fantasies, of course, are expressed in terms of this language, as is apparent from some of the contact ads presented above. It is important to note that fantasies are not unique, private, and idiosyncratic, but instead, involve *culturally general* resources—typifications of persons, of typical actions and situations, and so forth. Fantasies are part of the culture.

Summary and Conclusions

This paper represents an initial attempt to provide a theoretical structure for the sociological study of sadomasochism. Sadomasochistic behavior, like human behavior in general, is most fully understood within a social context. To understand "what is going on" within an S&M episode, one must know something about the culture of the group and how it defines and categorizes people and behavior. This is where frame analysis is helpful. Frames are central components of the culture of the group, through which its members interpret the world. To a great extent the frame itself is structured by the language of the group, which serves to explain to its members what is happening and to justify their desires, motives, and behavior. Frames tell people what is and what is not proper, acceptable, and possible within their world. They define and categorize for their members situations, settings, scenes, identities, roles, and relationships.

When people join sadomasochistic groups, or any other kind of group, they are taught not only frames, but also the conceptual tools or "keys" for defining, applying, transforming, and limiting them.

Frame analysis helps make sense of findings that might otherwise be difficult to explain. For example, the apparently puzzling existence in the S&M subculture of "dominant" women and "submissive" men when the larger society to which these individuals also belong prescribes aggressiveness for males and passivity for females may be explained in terms of make-believe, fantasy, and the theatrical frame. Lack of generalization into the larger world of roles and relationships developed within the sadomasochistic subworld is explained in terms of how behavior is "keyed."

A number of areas that have not been fully developed here could be profitably explored. For example, although we have attended to the structuring and limiting of S&M frames, we have not explored misframings, miskeyings, breaking frame, and other errors and their consequences for interactants. Hollander (1972), for instance, provides an example in which an S&M episode was miskeyed with disastrous results. Another issue for further exploration involves the ways in which the language of S&M structures the relations between participants in that world by building in notions of activity and passivity and tying these to particular roles in the interaction. The specific identities of people as "dominant" or "submissive," the ways in which they arrive at a recognition of these self-identities, and the stability of these orientations await investigation.[2]

Notes

1. "B&D" is Bondage and Discipline, which refers to controlling another person's behavior through physical restraints or bonds, or by verbal commands. Various punishments may be used to gain compliance.—Ed.

2. A number of these questions are addressed by other essays in this collection. For example, G. W. Levi Kamel develops a theoretical structure for analyzing the acquisition of a "leatherman" self-identity among homosexuals, and Kamel and Weinberg explore the development and practice of sadomasochistic identities as an interactive

process in "Diversity in Sadomasochism: Four S&M Careers." In this essay they give examples of the ways in which identities such as "dominant" and "submissive" evolve and are modified by the needs of one's partners.—Ed.

References

Buffalo Courier-Express, 1977. "2 homosexuals quizzed in 43 killings" (July 4).

Coburn, J. 1977. "S&M." *New Times* 8 (February 4): 43, 45–50.

Cohen, A. K. 1955. *Delinquent Boys: The Culture of the Gang.* Glencoe, Ill.: The Free Press.

DeLora, J. S., and C. A. B. Warren. 1977. *Understanding Sexual Interaction.* Boston: Houghton Mifflin Company.

Dietz, P. E. 1978. *Kotzwarraism: Sexual Induction of Cerebral Hypoxia.* Medical Criminology Research Center, McLean Hospital. (Unpublished manuscript.)

Footlick, J. K., and S. Smith. 1975. "Did the Bikers Do It?" *Newsweek* 85 (February 17): 63–64.

Gagnon, J. 1977. *Human Sexualities.* Glenview, Ill.: Scott, Foresman and Company.

Goffman, E. 1963. *Stigma: Notes on the Management of Spoiled Identity.* Englewood Cliffs, N. J.: Prentice-Hall.

Goffman, E. 1974. *Frame Analysis.* Cambridge, Mass.: Harvard University Press.

Halpern, B. 1977. "Spanks for the Memory." *Screw* 420 (March 21): 4–7.

Hollander, X. 1972. *The Happy Hooker.* New York: Dell.

Kaplan, A. 1964. *The Conduct of Inquiry.* San Francisco: Chandler Publishing Company.

Newsweek. 1966. "The Trial Begins." 67 (May 2): 34.

Pengelley, E. T. 1978. *Sex and Human Life,* 2d ed. Menlo Park, Calif.: Addison-Wesley Publishing Company.

Scott, M. B., and S. M. Lyman. 1968. "Accounts." *American Sociological Review* 33: 46–62.

Sykes, G., and D. Matza. 1957. "Techniques of Neutralization: A Theory of Delinquency." *American Sociological Review* 22: 664–70.

Sutherland, E. H., and D. R. Cressey. 1960. *Principles of Criminology,* 6th ed. New York: J. B. Lippincott Company.

Time. 1976. "Homosexuality: Gays on the March." 106 (September 8): 32–37, 43.

Von Cleef, M. 1971. *The House of Pain.* Secaucus, N. J.: Lyle Stuart.

Weinberg, T. S. 1976. *Becoming Homosexual: Self-discovery, Self-identity, and Self-maintenance.* Ph.D. diss., University of Connecticut.

Weinberg, T. S., and G. Falk. 1978. Sadists and Masochists: The Social Organization of Sexual Violence. Read before the Annual Meeting of the Society for the Study of Social Problems, San Francisco, Calif.

West C., and D. H. Zimmerman. 1977. "Women's Place in Everyday Talk: Reflections on Parent-Child Interaction." *Social Problems* 24: 521–29.

Pat Califia

A Secret Side of Lesbian Sexuality

The sexual closet is bigger than you think. By all rights, we shouldn't be here, but we are. It's obvious that conservative forces like organized religion, the police, and other agents of the tyrannical majority don't want sadomasochism to flourish anywhere, and sexually active women have always been a threat the system won't tolerate. But conservative gay liberationists and orthodox feminists are also embarrassed by kinky sexual subcultures (even if that's where they do their tricking). "We are just like heterosexuals (or men)," is their plea for integration, their way of whining for some of America's carbon monoxide pie. Drag queens, leathermen, rubber freaks, boy-lovers, girl-lovers, dyke sadomasochists, prostitutes, transsexuals—we make that plea sound like such a feeble lie. We are not like everyone else. And our difference is not created solely by oppression. It is a preference, a sexual preference.

This article is reprinted by permission of *The Advocate*, P.O. Box 5847, San Mateo, CA 94402. It originally appeared in Issue 287 (December 27, 1979) of *The Advocate*. Copyright © 1979 by L.P. Publications, Inc.

Lesbian S&M isn't terribly well-organized (yet). But in San Francisco, women can find partners and friends who will aid and abet them in pursuing the delights of dominance and submission. We don't have bars. We don't even have newspapers or magazines with sex ads. I sometimes think the gay subculture must have looked like this, when urbanization first started. Since our community consists of word-of-mouth and social networks, we have to work very hard to keep it going. It's a survival issue. If the arch-conformists with their cardboard cunts and angora wienies had their way, we wouldn't exist at all. As we become more visible, we encounter more hostility, more violence. This article is my way of refusing the narcotic of self-hatred. We must break out of the silence that persecution imposes on its victims.

I am a sadist. The polite term is "top," but I don't like to use it. It dilutes my image and my message. If someone wants to know about my sexuality, they can deal with me on my own terms. I don't particularly care to make it easy. S&M is scary. That's at least half its significance. We select the most frightening, disgusting, or unacceptable activities and transmute them into pleasure. We make use of all the forbidden symbols and all the disowned emotions. S&M is a deliberate, premeditated, erotic blasphemy. It is a form of sexual extremism and sexual dissent.

I identify more strongly as a sadomasochist than as a lesbian. I hang out in the gay community because that's where the sexual fringe starts to unravel. Most of my partners are women, but gender is not my boundary. I am limited by my own imagination, cruelty, and compassion, and by the greed and stamina of my partner's body. If I had a choice between being shipwrecked on a desert island with a vanilla lesbian and a hot male masochist, I'd pick the boy. This is the kind of sex I like—sex that tests physical limits within a context of polarized roles. It is the only kind of sex I am interested in having.

I am not typical of S&M lesbians, nor do I represent them. In fact, because I define myself as a sadist, I am atypical. Most S&M people *prefer* the submissive "bottom" or masochistic role. The bulk of the porn (erotic, psychoanalytic, and political) that gets written about S&M focuses on the masochist. People who do public speaking about S&M have told me they get a more sympathetic hearing if they identify as bottoms. This makes sense, in a twisted kind of way. The uninitiated associate masochism with incompetence, lack of assertiveness, and self-destruction. But sadism is associated with chainsaw murders. A fluffy-sweater type listening to a masochist may feel sorry for her, but she's terrified of me. I'm the one who is ostensibly responsible for manipulating or coercing the M into degradation—all 130 pounds 5' 2" of me. Therefore, my word is suspect. It is nevertheless true that my services are in demand, that I respect my partners' limits, and that both (or more) of us obtain great pleasure from a scene. I started exploring S&M as a bottom, and I still put my legs in the air now and then. I have never asked a submissive to do something I haven't or couldn't do.

In addition to being a sadist, I have a leather fetish. If I remember my Krafft-Ebing, that's another thing women aren't supposed to do. Oh, well. Despite the experts, seeing, smelling, or handling leather makes me cream. Every morning before I go out the door, I make a ritual out of putting on my leather jacket. The weight of it, settling on my shoulders, is reassuring. Once I zip it, turn the collar up, and cram my hands into the pockets, the jacket is my armor. It also puts me in danger when I wear it on the street by alerting the curious and the angry to my presence.

I get all kinds of different reactions. Voyeurs drool. Queer-baiting kids shout or throw bottles from their cars. Well-dressed hets,[1] secure in their privilege, give me the condescending smile of the genital dilettante. Some gay men are amused when they see me coming. They take me for a fag hag,[2] a mascot dressed up to avoid embarrassing my macho friends. Others are resentful. Leather is their province, and a cunt is not entitled to wear the insignia of a sadomasochist. They avoid my shadow. I might be menstruating and make their spears go dull. When I visit a dyke bar, the patrons take me for a member of that nearly-extinct species, the butch. Femmes under this misapprehension position themselves within my reach, signaling their availability, not bothering to actively pursue me. They seem to expect me to do everything a man would do, except knock them up. Given the fact that I prefer someone to come crawling and begging for my attention, and to work pretty damned hard before they get it, this strikes me as being very funny. In women's groups, the political clones, the Dworkinites,[3] see my studded belt and withdraw. I am obviously a sex pervert, and good, real true lesbians are not sex perverts. They are high priestesses of feminism, conjuring up the "wimmin's" revolution. As I understand it, after the wimmin's revolution, sex will consist of wimmin holding hands, taking their shirts off, and dancing in a circle. Then we will all fall asleep at exactly the same moment. If we didn't all fall asleep, something else might happen— something male-identified, objectifying, pornographic, noisy, and undignified. Something like an orgasm.

This is why they say leather is expensive. When I wear it, disdain, amusement, and the threat of violence follow me from my door to my destination and home again. Is it worth it? Can the sex be that good? When am I going to get to the point and tell you what we do?

I can smell your titillation. Well—since you want it so bad, I'll let you have a taste of it.

If I'm interested in someone, I call them up and ask them if they'd like to go out for dinner. I have never picked up a stranger in a bar. My partners are friends, women who strike up acquaintances with me because they've heard me talk about S&M, women I know from Samois.[4] (I also have a lover who is my slave. We enjoy conducting joint seductions or creating bizarre sexual adventures to tell each other about later.) If she agrees, I will tell her where and when to meet me. Over dinner, I begin to play doctor—Dr. Kinsey. I like to know when she started being sexual with other people, if and when she started masturbating, if and how she likes to have an orgasm, when she came out as a lesbian (if she has), and I give her similar information about me. Then I like to ask about her S&M fantasies and how much experience she has with acting them out. I also try to find out if she has any health problems (asthma, diabetes, etc.) that should limit play.

This conversation need not be clinical. It is not an interview—it is an interrogation. I am taking for granted my right to possess intimate information about my quarry. Giving me that information is the beginning of her submission. The sensations this creates are subtle, but we both begin to get turned on.

I will probably encourage her to get a little high. I don't like playing with women who are too stoned to feel what I am doing, nor do I want someone shedding inhibitions because of a chemical they've ingested. I prefer to deny a bottom any inhibitions and to take them away. However, I do like her to feel relaxed and somewhat vulnerable and suggestible.

If there's time, we may go to a bar. Socializing in gay men's leather bars is problematic for a lesbian. I prefer bars where I know some of the bartenders and patrons. I have rarely been refused admittance, but I have been made uncomfortable by men who felt I was an intruder. If there were women's bars that didn't make me feel even more unwelcome, I'd go there. Since I am a sadomasochist, I feel entitled to the space I take up in a men's bar. I sometimes wonder how many of the men exhibiting their leather in the light from the pinball machines go home and really work it out, and how many of them settle for fucking and sucking.

A leather bar provides a safe place to start establishing roles. I like to order my submissive to bring me a drink. She doesn't get a beer of her own. When she wants a drink, she asks me for one, and I pour it into her mouth while she kneels at my feet. I begin to handle her, appraising her flesh, correcting her posture, and fondling or exposing her so that she feels embarrassed and draws closer to me. I like to hear someone ask for mercy or protection. If she isn't already wearing a collar, I put one on her, and drag her over to a mirror—behind the bar, in the bathroom, on a wall—and make her look at it. I watch the response very carefully. I don't like women who collapse into passivity, whose bodies go limp and faces go blank. I want to see the confusion, the anger, the turn-on, the helplessness.

As soon as I am sure she is turned on (something that can be ascertained with the index finger if I can get her zipper down), I hustle her out of there. I especially like to put someone in handcuffs and lead them out on a leash.

This is one of the gifts I offer a submissive: the illusion of having no choice, the thrill of being taken.

The collar will keep her aroused until we reach my flat. I prefer to play in my space since it's set up for bondage and whipping. I will order her to stay two steps behind me, to reassure her that we really are going to do a scene. As soon as the door is locked behind us, I order her to strip. In my room, there is no such thing as casual nudity. When I take away someone's clothing, I am temporarily denying their humanity, with all its privileges and responsibilities.

Nudity can be taken a step further. The bottom can be shaved. A razor, passing over the skin, removes the pelt that warms and conceals. My lover/slave has her cunt shaved. It reminds her that I own her genitals, and reinforces her role as my child and property.

Shedding her clothes while I remain fully dressed is enough to shame and excite most bottoms. Once she is naked, I put her on the floor, and there she stays until I move her or raise her up. I stand over her, trail a riding crop down her spine, and tell her that she belongs underneath me. I talk about how good she's going to make my cunt feel and how strict I am going to be with her. I may allow her to embrace my boots. After delineating her responsibilities and cussing her out a little for being easy, I haul her up, slap her face, hold her head against my hip while I unzip, and let her feast on my clit.

I wonder if any man could understand how this act, receiving sexual service, feels to me. I was taught to dread sex, to fight it off, to provide it under duress or in exchange for romance and security. I was trained to take responsibility for other people's gratification and pretend pleasure when others pretend to have my pleasure in mind. It is shocking and profoundly satisfying to commit this piece of rebellion, to take pleasure exactly as I want it, to exact it like tribute. I need not pretend I enjoy a bottom's ministration if they are unskilled, nor do I need to be grateful.

I like to come before I do a scene because it takes the edge off my hunger. For the same reason, I don't like to play when I am stoned or drunk. I want to be in control. I need all my wits about me to outguess the bottom's needs and fears, take her out of herself, and bring her back. During the session, she will receive much more direct physical stimulation than I will. So I take what I need. From her mouth, she feeds me the energy I need to dominate and abuse her.

While I am getting off, I usually begin to fantasize about the woman on her knees. I visualize her in a certain position or a certain role. This fantasy is the seed that the whole scene sprouts from. When she's finished pleasing me, I order her to crawl onto my bed, which is on the floor, and I tie her up.

Bottoms tend to be anxious. Because there is a shortage of tops, they get used to playing all kinds of little psychological numbers on themselves to feel miserable and titillated. They also like to feel greedy and guilty, and get anxious about that. The bondage is reassurance. She can measure the intensity of my passion by the tightness of my knots. It also puts an end to bullshit speculation about whether I am doing this just because she likes it so much. I make sure there's no way she can get loose on her own. Restraint becomes security. She knows I want her. She knows I am in charge.

Being tied up is arousing, and I intensify this arousal by teasing her, playing with her breasts and clit, calling her nasty names. When she starts to squirm, I begin to rough her up a little, taking her to the edge of pain, the edge that melts and turns over into pleasure. I move from pinching her nipples to a pair of clamps that makes then ache and burn. I may put clips all over her breasts or on the labia. I will check her cunt to make sure it's still wet, and tell her how turned on she is, if she doesn't already know.

At some point, I will always use a whip. Some bottoms like to be whipped until they are bruised. Others find just the visual image exciting and may want to hear the sound of it whistling in the air or feel the handle moving in and out of them. A whip is a great way to get someone to be here now. They can't look away from it, and they can't think about anything else.

If the pain goes beyond a mild discomfort, the bottom will probably get scared. She will start to wonder, "Why am I doing this? Am I going to be able to take this?" There are many ways to get someone past this point. One is to ask her to take it for me because I need to watch her suffer. One is to administer a fixed number of blows as a punishment for some sexual offense. Another is to convince a bottom that they deserve the pain, and must endure it because they are "only" a slave. Pacing is essential. The sensations need to increase gradually. The particular implement involved may also be important. Some women who cannot tolerate whipping have a very high tolerance for other things—nipple play, hot wax, enemas, or verbal humiliation.

When I am playing bottom, I don't want pain or bondage for their own sake. I want to please. The top is my mistress. She has condescended to train me, and it is very important to me to deserve her attention. The basic dynamic of S&M is the power dichotomy, not pain. Handcuffs, dog collars, whips, kneeling, being bound, tit clamps, hot wax, enemas, penetration, and giving sexual service are all metaphors for the power imbalance. However, I must admit that I get bored pretty fast with a bottom who is not willing to take any pain.

The will to please is a bottom's source of pleasure, but it is also a source of danger. If the top's intentions are dishonorable (i.e., emotional sabotage) or her skill is faulty, the bottom is not safe when she yields. The primary point of competition among tops is to be emotionally and physically safe to play with, to be worthy of the gift of submission. Someone who makes mistakes gets a bad reputation very fast, and only inexperienced or foolish bottoms will go under for them.

Why would anyone want to be dominated, given the risks? Because it is a healing process. As a top, I find the old wounds and unappeased hunger. I nourish, I cleanse and close the wounds. I devise and mete out appropriate punishments for old, irrational sins. I trip the bottom up, I see her as she is, and I forgive her and turn her on and make her come, despite her unworthiness or self-hatred or fear. We are all afraid of losing, of being captured and defeated. I take the sting out of that fear. A good scene doesn't end with orgasm—it ends with catharsis.

I would never go back to tweaking tits and munching cunt in the dark, not after this. Two lovers sweating against each other, each struggling for her own goal, eyes blind to each other—how appalling, how deadly. I want to see and share in every sensation and emotion my partner experiences, and I want all of it to come from me. I don't want to leave anything out. The affronted modesty and the hostility are as important as the affection and lust.

The bottom must be my superior. She is the victim I present for the night's inspection. I derive an awful knowledge from each gasp, the tossing head, the blanching of her knuckles. In order to force her to lose control, I must unravel her defenses, breach her walls, and alternate subtlety and persuasion with brutality and violence. Playing a bottom who did not demand my respect and admiration would be like eating rotten fruit.

S&M is high technology sex. It is so time-consuming and absorbing that I have no desire to own anyone on a full-time basis. I am satisfied with their sexual submission. This is the difference between real slavery or exploitation and S&M. I am interested in something ephemeral, pleasure, not in economic control or forced reproduction.

This may be why S&M is so threatening to the established order, and why it is so heavily penalized and persecuted. S&M roles are not related to gender or sexual orientation or race or class. My own needs dictate which role I will adopt. Our political system cannot digest the concept of power unconnected to privilege. S&M recognizes the erotic underpinnings of our systems, and seeks to reclaim them. There's an enormous hard-on beneath the priest's robe, the cop's uniform, the president's business suit, the soldier's khakis. But that phallus is powerful only as long as it is concealed, elevated to the level of a symbol, never exposed or used in literal fucking. A cop with his hard-on sticking out can be punished, rejected, blown, or you can sit on it, but he is no longer a demi-god. In an S&M context, the uniforms and roles and dialogue become a parody of authority, a challenge to it, a recognition of its secret sexual nature.

Governments are based on sexual control. Any group of people who gain access to authoritarian power become accessories to that ideology. They begin to perpetuate and enforce sexual control. Women and gays who are hostile to other sexual minorities are siding with fascism. They don't want the uniforms to degenerate into drag—they want uniforms of their own.

As I write this, there is a case in Canada that will determine whether or not S&M sex between consenting adults can be legal. This case began when a gay male bathhouse that caters to an S&M clientele was raided. After that raid, a man in Toronto was busted for "keeping a common bawdy house." The "bawdy house" was a room in his apartment he had fixed up for S&M sex. Yet another man was busted for false imprisonment and aggravated assault. These charges stemmed from an S&M three-way.[5]

In San Francisco, months before Moscone and Milk were assassinated and the cops smashed into the Elephant Walk, half the leather bars in the Folsom Street area lost their liquor licenses due to police harassment. The Gay Freedom Day Parade Committee tried to pass a resolution that would bar leather and S&M regalia from the parade.

I don't know how long it will take for other S&M people to get as angry as I am. I don't know how long we will continue to work in gay organizations that patronize us and threaten us with expulsion if we don't keep quiet about our sexuality. I don't know how long we will continue to let women's groups who believe that S&M and pornography are the same thing and cause violence against women to go unchallenged because they are ostensibly feminist. I don't know how long we will continue to run our sex ads in magazines that feature judgmental, slanderous articles about us. I don't know how long we will continue to be harassed and assaulted or murdered on the street, or how long we will tolerate the fear of losing our apartments or being fired from our jobs or arrested for making the wrong kind of noise during some heavy sex.

I do know that whenever we start to get angry, walk out, and work for our own cause, it will be long overdue.

Notes

1. "Het," slang for heterosexual.—Ed.

2. "Fag hag," a heterosexual woman who associates extensively with male homosexuals.—Ed.

3. Dworkinites are followers of Andrea Dworkin, an activist in Women Against Pornography. She has often been criticized for what have been perceived as anti-male and anti-sexual attitudes.—Ed.

4.. SAMOIS is a support group for lesbians interested in S&M, located in the San Francisco Bay area.—Ed.

5. As of early 1983, a number of these cases were still slowly being processed through the courts. Jim Bartley, in an article entitled "Morality: Fishing for Victims," appearing in the January 1983 issue of *Body Politic* (Toronto's gay newspaper), notes that 90 percent of the cases have resulted in acquittal.—Ed.

James Myers

Nonmainstream Body Modification: Genital Piercing, Branding, Burning, and Cutting

The term *body modification* properly includes cosmetics, coiffure, ornamentation, adornment, tattooing, scarification, piercing, cutting, branding, and other procedures done mostly for aesthetic reasons. It is a phenomenon possibly as old as genus *Homo*, or at least as ancient as when an intelligent being looked down at some clay on the ground, daubed a patch of it on each cheek, and caught the pleasing reflection on the surface of a pond. Appropriate to my overall topic is Thevos's (1984) observation that a "self retouching impulse" distinguishes humans from other animals (p. 3).

At the outset, it is important to distinguish between the two main types of body modification: permanent (or irreversible) and temporary. Permanent modifications, such as tattooing, branding, scarification, and piercing, result in indelible markings on the surface of the body. With the exception of branding, these marks involve the application of sharp instruments to the skin.

James Myers, *Journal of Contemporary Ethnography* 21, no. 3, pp. 267–306, copyright © 1992 by Sage Publications, Inc. Reprinted by permission of Sage Publications, Inc.

Dental alterations, skull modeling, and modern plastic surgery are also forms of permanent body modification. Temporary modifications include body painting, cosmetics, hair styling, costume, ornamentation, and any other alteration that can be washed off, dusted away, or simply lifted off the body. This article focuses on permanent body modifications in contemporary United States, especially genital piercing, branding, and cutting.[1]

The literature of anthropology abounds with descriptive and analytical accounts of body modification among humans, but almost all of it emanates from people living or who had lived in the non-Western traditional societies of the world. From Mayan tongue piercing to Mandan flesh skewering, Ubangi lip stretching to Tiv scarification, there is a vast and incredibly varied body of literature that seeks to explain it all—anthropologically, psychologically, sociologically, and biologically. Curiously, very little research has been done on contemporary, nonmainstream American body modification. When one considers the huge amount of literature devoted to the subject among traditional non-Western peoples, this paucity of data becomes glaringly evident. For example, one of the best recent sources on body modification is Rubin's (1988) *Marks of Civilization*, but even in this excellent publication, most of the articles deal with tattoos and cicatrization and none are devoted to such contemporary Euro-American practices as multiple piercing, scarification, cutting, and branding.

That a tattoo renaissance has been occurring in the United States since the late 1960s is now quite evident in the popular media and to a growing extent in scholarly publications and papers presented at professional conferences (see especially Govenar 1977; Rubin 1988; Sanders 1986, 1988a, 1988b, 1989; St. Clair and Govenar 1981).[2] This void in the literature is probably due more to a simple lack of awareness of the practice than it is a lack of interest, as the population of people involved in multiple piercing, scarification, branding, and cutting is minuscule compared to tattooing. In addition, because the modification and/or jewelry involved typically creates even greater revulsion in the general public's eye than tattoos, much of the work is kept secret among recipients and their intimates.

My observations and conclusions regarding nonmainstream body modification run counter to the general public's assessment that people so involved are psychological misfits bent on disfigurement and self-mutilation. None of the people I interviewed, however deep and varied their involvement in body alteration, fit the standard medical models for "self-mutilation."

This article contains four major sections. First, I discuss the methods used and the population involved in the study. This section also includes some thoughts on the pleasures and problems of conducting fieldwork with nonmainstream body modifiers. Following this is a presentation of the ethnographic data, the largest portion of which is devoted to a description of my participant observation work with four different body modification workshops in San Francisco, California. The next section explores the motivation and rationale behind those who participate in body modification despite the physical pain involved and the stigma that American society attaches to the behavior. Finally, I conclude with some observations on the conventionality of the individuals in the study, an assessment that runs counter to the prevailing medical literature on the subject and the views held by the general American public. I also relate nonmainstream body modification to the worldwide practice of rites of passage and the rich body of ritual symbolism accompanying such rites.[3]

Method and Population

My original plan was to concentrate my research efforts on tattooing, but four months into the twenty-four-month study period, I shifted my focus almost entirely to piercing, cutting, burning, and branding. The change was brought about by my increasing awareness of the growing popularity of nonmainstream modification other than tattoos and the realization that research on the subject was scant. I was also intrigued by the deep feelings of revulsion and resentment held by mainstream American society against these forms of body modification.[4]

Using participant observation and interviews as primary data-gathering techniques, I involved myself in six workshops organized especially for the San Francisco SM (sadomasochist) community by Powerhouse (fictitious name), a San Francisco Bay area SM organization.[5] Tattoo and piercing studios were also a rich source of data, as was the Fifth Annual Living in Leather Convention held in Portland, Oregon in October 1990. I gathered additional data from a small but dedicated group of nonmainstream body modifiers at my university and the city in which it is located. Interviews with several medical specialists and an examination of pertinent medical literature provided an important perspective, as did solicited and unsolicited commentary from hundreds of mainstream society individuals who viewed my body modification slides and/or heard me lecture on the topic. Finally, chance encounters with devotees served to broaden my awareness and understanding of the various forms of nonmainstream body modification.

Entree to the workshops was of paramount importance to the study; thus early in the fieldwork, I contacted the primary organizer of Powerhouse and introduced myself as a straight, male anthropologist interested in attending the workshops in order to gather data on nonmainstream body modification for use in my university classroom and publication in a scholarly journal. Her response was immediate:

> Good God, yes! You're welcome to come. We need people to see that just because we're kinky doesn't mean we're crazy, too. You'll see people here with all kinds of sexual interests. We learn from each other and have a heckuva lot of fun while we're at it.

As is true for most ethnographic participant observation situations, the largest amount of my data from the workshops were gathered from observation. I participated in the true sense of the word on two occasions, once during a play piercing demonstration and again during a playing with fire demonstration.[6] The rest of my participation involved such typical "interested involvement" as mingling, asking questions as an audience member, introducing myself around, helping arrange chairs, setting up demonstration paraphernalia, taking photographs, conducting interviews, and generally lending a hand whenever possible. At the Living in Leather Convention in Portland, I was able to expand my involvement by showing my body modification slides to several people, attending parties, and helping out at the host organization's hospitality suite.

The population of body modifiers in my study included males and females, heterosexuals and homosexuals (lesbians and gays), bisexuals, and SMers. It is important to note that the single largest group was composed of SM homosexuals and bisexuals. Although this skewing likely resulted from my extended contact with the Powerhouse workshops and several SM body modifiers who I interviewed at the Living in Leather Convention in Portland, it is supported by a 1985 piercing profile of subscribers to *Piercing Fans International Quarterly* (Nichols 1985). The survey determined that 37 percent of the group was gay, 15 percent bisexual, and 57 percent involved in dominant-submissive play, a keystone of SM activity. Also of interest from the *PFIQ* profile, 83 percent had attended college, 24 percent had college degrees, and 33 percent had undertaken postgraduate study. Caucasians represented 93 percent of the survey.

Like any fieldwork, this research had its pleasant and difficult aspects. On the positive side was the subject matter itself. Body modification is inherently fascinating to human beings. In addition, there was the relative ease with which I was able to gather empirical data on the topic. The people I interviewed and observed were for the most part barely subdued exhibitionists who took joy in displaying and discussing their body and its alterations. This was especially true when a group was together and a sense of trust pervaded the room. On such occasions, an exuberant "show and tell" was the order of the day. To field-workers accustomed to tight-lipped, monosyllabic responses and other forms of "informant lockjaw" from people they are studying, and who have been advised on occasion what they could do with their camera, it should be understandable why it was a pleasure to work with this uninhibited, communicative population.[7]

Such rapport presupposes that an element of trust has been achieved between the field-worker and the individuals or group being studied. Many people who I interviewed were keenly aware that because mainstream society regarded them as deviants, there was a high probability that harm to themselves or their life-style was never far away. Thus interaction between the field-worker and the individuals being studied must occur early to establish the trust necessary to conduct a worthwhile study.

Naturally, there were dilemmas and problems, of which photography loomed the largest. Photography is a must in any discipline where the recording and analysis of visual data is important, but unfortunately it also has the capability of violating the personal world of those being studied. The agonizing dilemma in my use of the camera at workshops and with individual informants quickly became apparent to me. Body modification is a visually charged phenomenon that is by its very nature designed to be seen. The richest written description of a tattoo or piercing when compared to a photograph can only pale. I was always plagued by the nagging question, "Should I or shouldn't I?" Fortunately, many subjects made it easy for me by volunteering, "Would you like to take a picture?" Others queried me regarding the use of the photos and their concerns that they might appear in a newspaper or magazine. Some of them flatly said no, often with an apology and some such clarifying comment as, "My family lives in the area and they'd die if they knew what kind of scene I was into."

I always asked permission to take photos and tried to use common sense in determining whether or not a particular situation was appropriate for photography. For example, I did not take pictures during actual workshop demonstrations but did so only while people were socializing before and after each session.

I believe that, overall, my camera helped to reduce barriers between myself and my informants. Indeed, many people requested, and received from me, copies of photographs I had taken of them. This exchange served as a type of "cultural brokerage" and enhanced my rapport with several individuals. Still, I must confess that although I took hundreds of pictures during the fieldwork, I was never quite able to shake the uncomfortable feeling that I was intruding in someone's very personal life.

As always in fieldwork, there was the problem of assessing informant reliability. In the case of my SM body modifiers, this problem reached new heights for me because of their devotion to fantasy, imagination, and role-playing. For example, although role-playing in an SM relationship is usually reserved for a specific "scene," on a few occasions I encountered informants who cleverly remained in their contrived roles throughout my interview. If not detected, the ethnographic perils inherent in such a maneuver can be devastating. For example, I am reminded that it took me two weeks to discover that one Wolfgang Muller, who wore a heavy, shin-length Wehrmacht coat and spoke English with a thick German accent during my interview, was actually an American accountant from Oregon and not, as he led me to believe, an expatriated East German border guard who had recently immigrated to the United States after the Berlin Wall was razed.

Another difficult aspect of my research was continually having to affirm the legitimacy of my topic to campus colleagues. There were welcome exceptions, but most seemed to view my work as a thinly disguised voyeuristic adventure. I fared better within my own department, but even these culturally aware stalwarts were often incredulous and jokingly referred to me by such cute sobriquets as Dr. Kink or Professor Sleaze. For the most part, students were enthralled with the topic and, with mouths agape, viewed my slides with a mixture of curiosity and astonishment. However, some were less enthusiastic. During a one-semester period, the dean of my college received formal complaints from two students to the effect that I was showing pornography in class. In addition, a colleague for whom I guest-lectured was graced with a particularly nasty written assessment of my presentation. Of interest here is the zero number of complaints registered to me or anyone during my thirty-year period of discussing, semester after semester, similar forms of body modification in non-Western cultures. After listening to me ruminate on this problem, one of my anthropology graduate students offered a provocative observation, "As long as the tits and pricks being pierced are brown, OK—but if they're white, no way!"

Body Modification Workshops

Most of the ethnographic data in my study were derived from the body modification SM workshops I observed and the contacts I made while in attendance. These workshops were part of a series of continuing programs sponsored by Powerhouse and were designed to "enhance the SM experience."[8] Taught by individuals who were regarded as professional practitioners of various nonmainstream body modifications, the workshops were limited to a top enrollment of fifty people. The six workshops I attended were on male piercing, female piercing, branding and burning, cutting, play piercing, and playing with fire.[9] The audience at each workshop was markedly homogeneous. With the exception of myself and perhaps a half-dozen others, each session was typically attended by SM-oriented lesbians, gays, and bisexuals. Participants ranged in age from their late teens to their late fifties, with most attendees in their mid-twenties and thirties. Leather was predominant—jackets, trousers, skirts, chaps, trucker's caps, gloves, boots, arm bands, wrist bands, and gauntlets. Heavily laden key rings, hunting knives in leather scabbards, slave collars, and T-shirts with sexual preference messages were also omnipresent. Tattoos, lip and nasal septum piercings, and multiple pierced ears were quickly visible, whereas more intimate piercings, such as nipple, navel, and genital would become evident as the workshops proceeded. It is fair to say that the groups would have attracted some attention were they to have gathered in a suburban shopping mall.

The four workshops described here were held on Saturday afternoons in an upstairs room of a liberal church in San Francisco.[10] Two other workshops I attended but do not describe in this article were conducted in a small room above a popular San Francisco gay bar.

Male Piercing

The first workshop in the series was on male piercing. Jim Ward, the teacher, was the president of Gauntlet, Inc., one of the few firms in the world that manufactures nonmainstream pierce-wear. Recognized as a "master piercer," Ward has been piercing since the mid-1970s and has estimated that he has done 15,000 piercings in the fourteen years between 1975 and 1989. He is also the editor and publisher of *Piercing Fans International Quarterly* (*PFIQ*), a successful glossy publication devoted exclusively to the subject of piercing (see appendix for descriptions of piercings, both male and female).

Ward arrived at the workshop early to set up his piercing equipment and a massage table that would serve as a piercing couch. He was wearing Levi's, a studded belt, black boots, and a black T-shirt that had the logo "Modern Primitives" (see Vale and Juno 1989) printed above twelve white-bordered rectangles, each of which contained a graphic drawing of one of the most popular genital piercings. Ward's lover and assistant set out several jewelry display cases and arranged chairs for the audience. He had multiple ear piercings, a bonelike tusk in his nasal septum, and a Gauntlet button on his T-shirt that proclaimed "We've got what it takes to fill your hole."

Ward's popularity and fame were evident as several arrivees paid their respect by shaking his hand or hugging and kissing him. Even though the workshop was on male piercing, one third of the audience was women, a crossing-over evident at each of the workshops regardless of the gender-specific body modification being highlighted. Ward welcomed the group, confirmed that his prearranged volunteers were present, and began his discussion of male piercing. It was evident that he had been through the routine many times, which he had, both before live audiences and in his continuing series in *PFIQ*, "Piercing With a Pro." His presentation was divided into halves, the first of which was a general discussion of the topic, or as he said, "the ins and outs of piercings," and the second consisting of actual demonstrations. As was true of each of the Powerhouse workshops, there was much emphasis on safety, cleanliness, sterilization, and proper hygiene after the procedure. Assuming that most of his audience was already involved in or at least aware of piercing, Ward dispensed without definition such esoteric piercing terminology as ampallang, dydoe, frenum, Prince Albert, guiche, and so on. Questions were asked about autoclave temperatures, rubber gloves, anesthetics, antiseptics, play piercing versus permanent piercing, the dangers of AIDS and hepatitis, body rejection, jewelry selection, and the like.

During the break, I asked Ward about his own piercings:

Well, you can see them in my ear lobe and tragus, but I also have a Prince Albert in my cock and a nipple ring on each tit. Oh, I've got a guiche with a piece of cord in it, too. I'm wearing all that stuff right now. I've been piercing myself for twenty years, but I don't wear jewelry in most of the holes. I travel all over the country, and I can tell you it's a real mind-fuck to get on an airplane and sit next to some hunk knowing you've got all this sexy stuff on.

I also talked with an audience member who was not interested in getting pierced but wanted to see what the attraction was for his pierced friends:

I don't feel the need to get pierced. Actually, I'm deathly afraid of needles. I don't think I have to look like a pin cushion in order to look sexy. When I'm out cruising I might stuff my balls through a coupla cock rings. Gives me a great feeling and enough basket to turn a few heads. Best of all, no artificial holes in my body to get infected.

Ward's first volunteer after the break was a leather-clad male who wanted his left nipple repierced. He sat shirtless on the table as his companion offered him a reassuring hug. Ward examined the nipple and told the group the scar tissue from the previous piercing would make this one more difficult. He also took advantage of the audience's concern to note the difference between pain and sensation in piercing and that he preferred the latter term to best describe the feeling. The volunteer's facial expression gave the impression that he had some doubts about Ward's evaluation. Before starting the piercing, Ward summoned his second volunteer and explained to the group that before he did the nipple job he needed to prep Number 2 for his forthcoming Prince Albert, a procedure that requires the application of a local anesthetic because the needle pierces the urethra, a particularly sensitive area. Number 2 dropped his leather trousers to his ankles, and Ward casually tamped a xylacane-coated cotton swab into the urethra about one inch. A male in the audience teased, "I bet he wishes there wasn't any anesthetic on that Q-tip.®" Laughter. Ward directed the volunteer to step over to one side of the room and wait for the anesthetic to numb the area. The volunteer, leather trousers still at his ankles and undershorts dropped below his knees, hopped over to the wall where he waited patiently, with the Q-tip® jauntily protruding from the tip of his penis.

Ward returned to the first volunteer and spent several moments discussing different types of male nipples and the particular piercing technique warranted by each. Then he scrubbed the volunteer's nipple with Hibiclens and Betadine, marked each side of the nipple with a dot to guide the needle path, clamped a Pennington forceps on the nipple to keep it from retracting and to afford better manageability, and expertly pushed a needle through the guide dots. An audible sharp gasp and a rigid tensing of the volunteer's body confirmed Ward's earlier comment about the likelihood of tougher tissue in repiercings. There was an immediate sigh of relief from the group accompanied by applause and congratulatory whoops. One end of the jewelry was used to push the needle the rest of the way through the nipple, thus resulting in the needle being expulsed and the jewelry attached in one continuous movement. The entire procedure had taken less than three minutes.

The second volunteer was invited back to the table, Q-tip® still in place as he waddled across the room. Ward had him sit on the table, then decided that it would be better if he stood on the table. There was some concern in the group about this stance, as the volunteer was visibly trembling, a circumstance that was all the more worrisome because the table itself began to shake. It was not clear whether the bare-legged volunteer was simply cold or whether he was suffering from pre-op jitters. Nevertheless, Number 2 balanced precariously atop the uncertain table while Ward, who had now gained an eye-level view of his work site, examined the about-to-be-pierced penis with his eyes and his fingers. As he worked, Ward maintained a running commentary on the history of the Prince Albert, noting that "it was originally designed to tether the penis to either the right or left pant leg for a neater looking appearance, but now it's strictly erotic." After completing the usual prepping around the piercing area, he deftly pushed the needle into the underside of the penis just behind the head, into the urethra, up toward the tip of the penis and the still lodged Q-tip®. As he pushed, the Q-tip® suddenly popped out of the urethra—"a sure sign I'm on course"—followed by the tip of the gleaming needle. The volunteer gazed warily down at the sight while being steadied by a friend. Applause and cheers. The jewelry was attached and Number 2 was eased down from the table. Still shaking, he pulled up his shorts and trousers. Ward peeled off his rubber gloves and disposed of them while discussing his thoughts on abstinence during the healing process.

The third volunteer was to receive a dydoe, a piercing that would pass through both sides of the upper edge of the glans. This volunteer, in his late forties, removed his trousers and undershorts and stretched out calmly on the table. With more than two hours of discussion and demonstrations behind him, Ward was now much quieter. The usual preliminaries were undertaken while the volunteer chattered about his piercing history. The group was only mildly interested in the disclosures, but full attention resumed when Ward began the actual piercing. As with the first two volunteers, this one emitted a controlled but audible gasp, then relaxed. The jewelry was attached and the volunteer hopped off the table and dressed while the group applauded. Later, this person expressed his feelings about piercing to me:

> I like the jewelry very much, but the real turn-on comes from having my body penetrated. Everytime I see that sharp, shiny needle heading towards my flesh I know I'm going to get either a dick orgasm or a head orgasm or maybe both.[11]

Several of the audience congratulated the new piercees and expressed their appreciation to Jim Ward. The first workshop was over.

Branding and Burning

The second workshop of the series was devoted to branding and burning and was taught by Fakir Musafer. Musafer, who pierced his own penis at age thirteen, was fifty-eight years old at the time of the workshop. Recognized by many as the doyen of "modern primitivism" in the United States, there is little in the practice of body modification and "body play" that he has not experienced on his own body. He has been tattooed, burned, cut, pierced, skewered, and electrically shocked. He has fasted, deprived himself of sleep, rolled on beds of thorns, and constricted and compressed various parts of his body with belts and corsets. He has also gilded, flagellated, punctured, and manacled himself. In addition to frequently suspending himself with fleshhooks à la the Sun Dance, he has reclined on a bed of nails or blades, "negated" his scrotum and penis by sealing them in plaster, and conversely "enhanced" the same by such practices as scrotum enlargement and penis elongation (a procedure accomplished by regular stretch workouts with three-pound weights, or, what he refers to as "rock on a cock" exercises). His fame continues to spread in the United States and abroad through his continuing involvement with Jim Ward's *PFIQ* and the release of "Dances Sacred and Profane," a widely distributed videotape that highlights his Sun Dance ritual. Musafer undoubtedly represents the distant end on any scale of contemporary nonmainstream body modifiers, the great percentage of whom are content with their tattoos and/or multiple piercings.

Musafer arrived thirty minutes before the start of the workshop. He was wearing a black T-shirt and baggy khaki cotton trousers with large flapped mid-leg pockets. Puffing on a cigarette, his hair dyed sable brown, and bereft of any visible piercing jewelry, he looked like any other middle-aged ad executive enjoying his weekend. I volunteered to help him unload his van. The contents of the box I carried up the stairs vaguely hinted of his workshop's topic—acetylene torch, metal snips, needle-nose pliers, wire, matches, incense sticks, candles, several strips of copper and tin, mirror, two potatoes, and various other oddities.

Like Jim Ward at the previous workshop, Musafer was hugged and kissed by many arrivees. And, as in all the workshops, a spirit of *bon homie* prevailed as arriving couples and singles of both sexes hugged and kissed acquaintances, chatted amiably with others, and shared their latest body art. A few moments before the starting time, Musafer shed his T-shirt, revealing a small ring in each nipple. He removed the rings and deftly replaced them with hollow metal tubes, each, according to his admission, ⅞ of an inch in diameter by 1 inch in length. Then he quickly inserted white teflon tubes through the holes on each side of his chest that had been created several years earlier for his Sun Dance hooks. Each tube was about the size of a king-sized cigarette and ran vertically through the flesh behind each nipple. Finally he reached into a pocket and pulled out a large nasal septum ring, which, with the aid of an audience member, was installed in his nose. He pulled his T-shirt back on and commented, "A-h-h, that's more like it!" Now, with open arms he welcomed everyone.

"The Fakir," as he frequently refers to himself, is an old pro at this sort of presentation and glibly but knowledgeably discussed his first topic of the day: branding. With the aid of an easel and predrawn charts, we learned about technique ("Don't go too deep, you're not doing a 'Mighty Dog' brand"), patterns ("The simpler the better"), important reminders ("Remember, each mark in the final scar will be two to four times thicker than the original imprint"), desirable locations ("The flatter the surface the better. Try to stick with the chest, back, tummy, thighs, butt, leg, upper arm"), and tools and materials and where to get them.

A prearranged volunteer indicated a preference for a 2-inch skull to be branded on the calf of her left leg. She reclined on the table with her skirt pulled up over her knees and her left leg extended toward Musafer's work site. A previously drawn pattern was transferred onto her left calf. As we watched, he fashioned the skull shape out of a strip of metal cut from a coffee can and showed us how to heat and apply the brand. Holding the brand in his needle-nosed pliers, he heated it in the acetylene torch until it was red hot, then quickly applied it to a piece of cardboard to check the design's appearance. Musafer also cut a potato in half and applied the reheated brand to the cut surface, noting that this was a good way for beginners to practice depth control before doing the real thing on human skin. The volunteer, a professional piercer and cutter in her early thirties, laughed with the audience as the potato hissed and smoked from Musafer's strike. "The Fakir" was now ready and alerted his client. The brand was heated, precisely positioned over the desired part of the pattern, and struck. There was an immediate hiss and a crackling sound, followed by a wisp of smoke and the odor of scorched flesh. The volunteer scarcely twitched. Musafer examined his first strike and proceeded to do six more to finish the skull, complete with stylized eyes, mouth, and teeth. The only time the volunteer reacted to the hot brand, and intensively so, was when Musafer inadvertently brushed the edge of her left foot with a "cooled" brand as he returned it to the torch for renewed heating. Musafer rubbed some Vaseline on the brand and the foot burn, and the volunteer sat up and put her low-cut boot back on. The audience applauded.

Musafer's next demonstration was on burning.[12] Displaying a row of seven or eight self-imposed circular burns on the front of his right thigh, each about the size of a penny and resembling inoculation scars, he discussed different types of burnings ("Cigarette burns are nasty but nice"), and techniques to cause them ("I prefer incense sticks because they work real well and smell so delightful during the burn"). There was no prearranged volunteer for burning, but a woman in her early twenties volunteered from the audience. Her friends cheered her as she removed her Levi's and sat on the table. Musafer touched her gently on the legs and softly said, "You are giving your flesh to the gods." He also instructed her on the importance of deep breathing and visualization as he glued a 3-inch length of incense stick to her left thigh and lit it. Within four or five minutes, the stick had burned down to skin level and extinguished itself. Although the stick was slightly less than a pencil in diameter, the circular burn mark quickly expanded to the penny sized marks I had viewed earlier on Musafer's thigh. Throughout the burning, the volunteer kept her eyes tightly closed and followed Musafer's instructions on deep breathing. She now opened her eyes and the audience applauded. Several of the audience members came up to where she was sitting and examined the burn, while one of her friends asked Musafer for some extra incense sticks to take home. Musafer doled out some sticks and jokingly admonished, "Watch it, this stuff is catching!" Many chuckles. Musafer responded to several last-minute questions while packing up his paraphernalia. This workshop had ended.

Female Piercing

The female piercing workshop was taught by Raelynn Gallina, a woman recognized throughout the Bay Area as a professional "total body" piercer. In addition to her popularity as a piercer and cutter (some of her clients glowingly refer to her as "Queen of the Blood Sports"), Raelynn is a successful designer and manufacturer of jewelry. Although she pierces males ("above the navel only"), the greatest proportion of her clientele is female, most of whom are, like herself, lesbian. She had been piercing for seven years at the time of the workshop. Two-thirds of the workshop's audience of forty-five people were women, all but a few of whom were lesbians involved in sadomasochism. Most of the men present were gay SMers. Raelynn announced that she had four volunteers for the afternoon and would pierce a nipple, a clitoris hood, an inner labia, and a nasal septum.

The first half of the workshop was devoted to a "do it yourself" clinic on technique, tools, antiseptics, and various dos and don'ts and ended with the admonition that it was safer and better to be pierced by a pro:

> I get a lot of people who want me to fix up their bungled piercings. Usually turns out they were heavy into a torrid scene when someone says, "Heh! Wouldn't it be hot if we pierced each other!" All I'm saying is if you do get carried away, make sure you know what you're doing.

After the break, Raelynn's spiritual-psychological bent revealed itself as she emphasized the importance of centering, grounding, visualization, client-practitioner compatibility, and the relationship between individual personality and type of piercing jewelry to be worn. She later commented to me:

> Piercing is really a rite of passage. Maybe a woman is an incest victim and wants to reclaim her body. Maybe she just wants to validate some important time in her life. That's why I like to have a ceremony to go along with my piercing and why I do it

in a temple—my home. Most of my clientele are bright, sensitive women. It's not as if a bunch of "diesel dykes" are busting into my place to prove how tough they are by getting their boobs punched through with needles.

Raelynn's first volunteer was an achondroplastic dwarf in her thirties. Dressed in leather trousers and field boots, it was obvious that she was extremely popular with many in the group. At least three different women lifted her up and danced merrily around with her in their arms during the break, while numerous others bent down to kiss her on the cheeks or lips. As Raelynn described the nipple piercing she was about to perform, the volunteer peeled off her blouse and climbed up on a long-legged director's chair. Clearly visible across her left breast in what appeared to be a recent cutting were the words "The bottom from Hell." There was much laughter, expressions of encouragement, and joking about anticipated pain, needles, second doubts, and the like. Raelynn scrubbed the volunteer's left breast and nipple with Hibiclens, applied a good coating of Betadine, and clamped a Pennington forceps on the nipple. The exact penetration and exit points for the needle were marked with a pen, and Raelynn quickly and expertly forced a needle through the nipple and into a small cork at the exit point. The forceps were removed, and a gold ring was inserted in the place of the needle. The only sign of pain from the volunteer was a short gasp as the needle pierced the nipple. As in the previous piercing procedures, there was a collective sigh of relief from the group, followed by applause and various congratulatory remarks. The volunteer climbed down from her perch and hugged Raelynn around the hips. Raelynn scooped her up, returned the hug, and kissed her.

By the time the first volunteer had put her blouse back on, the second volunteer had already removed her jeans and underpants and was sitting on the chair. In her mid-twenties, this volunteer would receive a clitoris hood piercing and jewelry. During most of the procedure, she held a hand mirror over her pubic area to better monitor the procedure. Raelynn advised the client to close her eyes and visualize the process. The piercing and jewelry attachment was completed within three minutes, again with the client showing minimal reaction to the actual piercing. As the volunteer pulled her tight jeans on, Raelynn reminded the group that it was important to wear loose-fitting clothes when getting a genital piercing.

The third volunteer, in her mid-twenties, had spent the first half of the workshop curled up in the laps of three different women. She removed her cotton skirt and hopped onto the chair. Pantyless and clean-shaven, two labia rings and a clitoris hood ring were easily visible. Raelynn announced that this client would be getting a third labia ring today and with a theatrical leer, added, "And she has asked me to do it real-l-l slow and with a twist." The audience responded with mock moaning and various teasing expressions. While Raelynn talked about genital piercing in general, the client sat spread-legged and observed with the hand mirror her present labia piercings and jewelry. Raelynn noted that a clamp was not usually needed for labia piercings and started the procedure. An audible intake of air and a slight tensing of the body were the only signs that the needle had pierced the flesh. The jewelry was quickly attached and the usual applause delivered.

I was unable to remain for the last piercing of the session, a nasal septum procedure through the nose of the first volunteer.

Cutting

Raelynn was also the teacher for the workshop on cutting. She had arrived in the room an hour before the scheduled starting time to set up her equipment and a videocamera. As people entered the room, she greeted them, occasionally examining a piercing or cutting that she had apparently performed at a previous occasion. By the starting time, forty-three people had arrived and there was the usual happy buzz of chatter. Three-fourths of the group were women, most of whom were wearing leather. As in the other workshops, the majority of the group members were gay and lesbian. Couples held hands, snuggled, kissed, and engaged in animated conversations. Raelynn sat on a table with knees crossed and officially greeted everyone. Although she welcomed the group by saying, "Hello fellow blood sluts," and there was a button attached to her equipment case that read "I'm hungry for your blood," she quickly stated she does her cutting for aesthetic reasons and not just for the joy of blood. Some of the audience responded in unison, "O-h-h, su-u-re!" She told the group she had been cutting for approximately 8 years and that she got her start while "caught up in some heavy SM scenes."

During the 2½-hour workshop, she discussed where cuttings should be done on the body ("Fleshy areas like the butt, thighs, back—not on the neck, joints, places where there are veins"), cleanliness ("Cutting is a clean procedure, not a sterile one"), use of rubber gloves, and concern about AIDS and hepatitis, depth of cut, design, tools, and various other bits of information regarding her subject. She also distinguished between her style of cutting and the types of scarification and cicatrization done in several preliterate populations of the world.

After a short break, Rosie, a prearranged volunteer in her forties, stripped to the waist to receive her cutting. She and Raelynn had decided earlier on a design that consisted of a pattern of stylized animal scales in a triangular shape. The design was large and would be cut into the upper left area of the back near the shoulder blade. Raelynn scrubbed Rosie's back with the usual antiseptics, dried it off, and covered the area with stick deodorant to facilitate the transfer of the design. Using a No. 15 disposable scalpel ("Toss it after it's been used"), she started her first incision. As she cut, she explained that cutting was not really a painful procedure because of the sharp scalpel and the shallow cuts. Someone in the group wondered aloud, "Is it bleeding yet?" to which someone else reported, "I certainly hope so!" Raelynn also urged would-be cutters to remember to start cutting at the bottom of the design so that the dripping blood would not wash away the uncut design. Both the cutter and the client were obviously moved by the procedure. Daubing away some blood, Raelynn told the group, "Once you start cutting someone, you get a very high, heady experience." Rosie, her eyes closed and mouth sensuously open, emitted several soft sighs during the ten-minute procedure. At one point, Rosie squeezed her companion's hand and whispered, "This is intense, wonderfully intense."

When the cutting was completed, Raelynn blotted the design several times to soak up the still bleeding incisions. Rosie was alerted to brace herself for the alcohol rinsings, which were done several times over the cutting. A towel around Rosie's waist kept the alcohol from dribbling further down her body. Raelynn then ignited a fresh rinsing of alcohol with her cigarette lighter. A loud poof was heard, and a bluish flame danced across the entire left side of Rosie's back. The flame was quickly doused as Raelynn announced, "Rosie asked me to do that because she's into fire." Referred to as "slash and burn" by Raelynn, the fire event was repeated two more times as the audience oohed and aahed. Finally, Raelynn rubbed black ink over the entire design and the wound was covered with a protective surgical wrap. In a few days, the excess ink would be scrubbed away, leaving the lines of the cutting colored black.

Kay, the second prearranged volunteer, wanted the fish cutting already on her back touched up. The original cutting had been done by Raelynn nine months earlier, and although the design was still easily discernible, Kay liked the idea of having it redone. Raelynn prepared the area, unpackaged a new scalpel, and recut the design in less than ten minutes. No ink was rubbed into the wound as Kay preferred the natural look.

Raelynn ended the workshop with a discussion of different body reactions to cutting, explaining that some people scarred nicely, well enough that there was no evidence of any cutting, whereas some keloided into large amorphous bumps.

While people were socializing after the session, I talked with a woman I recognized from earlier workshops. She told me Raelynn had pierced her labia, navel, and both nipples. She also compared Fakir Musafer and Jim Ward unfavorably with Raelynn:

> Those guys are out on the edge! They're an embarrassment. I mean, bones through the noses, the branding, the fleshhooks, the pain. You heard them—"If a client is in pain, you just keep on pushing and jabbing. It'll be over before you know it." Raelynn is great because she is gentle and looks for any special aspects of your personality that will help her do a better piercing or cutting.

Motivation and Rationale

Why do certain people in American society involve themselves in nonmainstream body modification? Considering the physical pain and the stigma attached to the behavior, what is the lure? Seeking answers to why people involve themselves in a given behavior is the life blood of the social sciences, but I learned early in my fieldwork that introducing the "why" question was a turn-off for some people and as such threatened rapport. As one person explained to me,

> I get tired of people asking me why I do it. They always get that dumb creaked-out look on their face when they see someone with a nose ring, or maybe they've heard that the office receptionist had her clit pierced and they can hardly wait to ask her why. Unless you've thought seriously of doing it, don't come around and ask why we do it.

Armed with this cautionary advice, I let people choose their own moment to express their thoughts on what motivated them. Fortunately, most of my informants volunteered their feelings without my having to ask them. Not surprising, there are no clear-cut, monolithic answers to the question. The reasons why people are motivated to have their bodies altered are extremely diverse as are the attempts of scholars to account for the behavior.[13]

The responses I received allowed me to construct several categories of individuals based on their stated motivation and rationale for being attracted to nonmainstream body modification.[14] A brief analytical commentary follows each category.

Sexual Enhancement

> A dick without a ring is like a sausage without spice. . . . Oh yes, just the slightest tug on any jewelry I'm wearing puts me on cloud nine. . . . My labia piercings look good, but it's my clit piercing that makes sex infinitely better. . . . The weight of the two rings on my clit always puts me in the mood for sex. . . . If all this stuff I'm wearing didn't make fucking better, I wouldn't be wearing it.

Sexual enhancement proved to be one of the most compelling reasons behind people's desire to alter their bodies. Even though sexual enhancement is presented here as a discrete motive, it cut across and joined with all eight categories. Thus whatever the motivational category, there was typically a sexual interest lurking somewhere behind the individuals' decisions to alter their bodies.

Although the high number of sadomasochists in the study population may be a skewing factor (one doesn't have to be around SMers long before realizing that sex is an all-consuming interest), it is clear that sexual enhancement was also a primary motive for the "vanillas" (non-SMers). Indeed, a perusal of the "Letters to the Editor" section of *Piercing Fans International Quarterly* confirms the sexual enhancement motive, regardless of the letter writer's sexual preference and practices. Vale and Juno's (1989) *Modern Primitives* contains interviews with several piercers, branders, and burners, most of whom identify sex as a prominent motivating factor among their recipients.

Jim Ward remarked that 90 percent of modern people are inspired to get a genital piercing so as to enhance their enjoyment of sex. "This is the primary reason—it definitely takes sex up a higher octave" (Vale and Juno 1989, p. 161).

The most commonly expressed belief about the sexual value of genital piercings and erotic jewelry is that they provide the wearer constant stimulation. Sheree Rose, a Los Angeles photographer active in West Coast tattoo and piercing communities, offered her feelings on the subject in Vale and Juno's (1989) *Modern Primitives*:

> You feel stimulation all the time. Those of us who like vibrators find it's incredible because you put the vibrator on the metal and the metal starts vibrating and—it just blows you away. (p. 110)

A married, heterosexual female in her mid-thirties told me,

> They feel wonderful. Just the feeling of that metal in my skin keeps me constantly aroused. It's like a little buzz in my body all the time.

In referring to the sexual value of his "ball weights" (not a piercing but stainless steel rings through which one pushes his scrotum so that the weight on the rings press down on the testicles), British body modifier Genesis P-Orridge observed in *Modern Primitives* (Vale and Juno 1989),

> once it's on, it feels like having your balls licked and sucked and being played with by someone's hand. . . .If someone pulls up on your cock, this weight pulls down on your balls, so you get this incredible interplay of up-and-down. You tend to have a semi-hard-on all the time when you wear them. (p. 177)

In addition to the basic "turn on" of simply having the piercing and jewelry in place, myriad manipulations and tricks are available to resourceful individuals and their partners. For example, depending on the type of jewelry and its location, it may be tugged, stroked, rotated, pushed, or bedecked with sundry devices of either an ornamental or functional nature. Certain piercings and jewelry may be used as tethering points for bondage enthusiasts. A chain or cord connected to one or several pieces of piercing jewelry presents numerous erotic possibilities: A strategic chain tug during sex may intensify pleasure or delay orgasm; a continuous network of delicate chains may interconnect several piercings on an individual (e.g., ears, nipples, navel, and labia), thus maximizing the number of erogenous zones that may be stimulated with a single pull; in an SM scene, a chain or cord may be attached to a slave's penis piercing or labia ring, allowing the master to "take the reins."

There is much discussion (and often spirited disagreement) among genital piercers as to which partner derives benefit during intercourse from a given piercing. Ostensibly, the ampallang (horizontal piercing through the penis head) favors the insertee; the apadravya (similar to ampallang, but the piercing runs vertically through the penis head) is commonly believed to increase sensation for both partners during intercourse; the Prince Albert (piercing through the urethra at the base of the penis head) is said to enhance pleasure for the wearer; labia and clitoris piercings are regarded as primarily beneficial to the wearer but also capable of intensifying a partner's pleasure.

Some individuals opt for piercings and jewelry that temporarily prohibit sex. A ring through the foreskin or a ring connecting the labia majora are examples of contemporary piercings that prevent sexual intercourse. Although most "chastity" piercing in the United States today are done for fantasy and/or erotic reasons, Jim Ward's exotic jewelry firm, Gauntlet, does a brisk business in manufacturing two types of rustless locks designed for fitting on genitalia: a purely decorative model called "The Imposter" and a functional version that requires a key. For the serious chastity-minded individual, a device called a Franey cage is available. The Franey cage involves two piercings, one at the base of the penis and the other through frenum, the effect of which even prohibits masturbation.

Piercing devotees believe that one's imagination and resourcefulness are the only limitations to the various sexual pleasures that may be derived from piercing.

Pain

> Anything as good as this has got to hurt—that's the icing on
> the cake. . . . All my little baubles are pretty, but the real head
> trip is anticipating the delicious pain that got them there. . . .Of
> course it's painful! Why else would Darcy want me to get
> pierced? . . . I look forward to the pain because it keeps my
> mind on the importance of what's happening to my body.

It would be incorrect to conclude that the SMers as a group
were lured to nonmainstream body modification solely because
of the likelihood of pain. Indeed, many SMers do not regard pain
as necessary for their masochistic experience.

After observing how the tattooees in his study stoically
accepted pain while receiving their tattoos, Sanders (1988b) concluded that it was difficult not to see the "ritualized initiatory
aspects" of tattooing (see also St. Clair and Govenar 1981). The
same logic may be extended to the nonmainstream body modifiers in my study. By identifying the body modification event as
an initiatory event, or a rite of passage, the importance of pain in
the process becomes readily evident.

Cross-cultural ethnographic literature has long recognized
pain as an essential element in rites of passage (e.g., Brain 1979;
Brown 1963; Ebin 1979; Gould 1968; Trigger 1969; Van Gennep
1960). Recognizing the process of inflicting and receiving pain in
public as part and parcel of a rite of passage ceremony, Bilmes
and Howard (1980) concluded that such ceremonies represent
ingeniously constructed cultural dramas involving three classes
of participants—inflictor, victim (initiate), and audience.
Although Bilmes and Howard supported their argument with
non-Western examples of ritual pain infliction, their rite-of-pas-
sage-as-cultural-drama thesis is particularly relevant to understanding the role of pain in body modification in contemporary
United States. For example, all three classes of participants were
evident in the piercing, branding, burning, and cutting events I
observed. The inflictor reigned supreme during a given body
modification drama, not only as the skilled practitioner who per-

formed the modification but as a model representative of the cadre of people who already possess some form of nonmainstream modification. The victim (or initiate) was the sine qua non of each event, having decided to endure the pain in order to become incorporated into the aspired ranks of body modifiers. As in all rites of passage, the initiate's comportment while undergoing pain is of paramount importance. The third class of participants, the audience, is also critical in the drama. Because a change of status frequently underlies a rite of passage ceremony, it is important that the drama be acknowledged by others. Sanders (1988b) observed that 69 percent of the tattooees in his study received their first tattoo with an audience of family or friends. Having witnesses enhances and validates one's transformation into the desired status, either as a first-timer or a repeating enthusiast. As Wickland and Gollwitzer (1982) pointed out, the acquisition of identity requires social reality—in other words, an audience (also see Gollwitzer 1986).

Thus pain, like sexual enhancement, was an underlying theme that was never far from the minds of those involved in the process. Although only a few individuals in the study stated that pain was a primary motive, everyone, SM or not, recognized its inevitability and importance, and greeted it with a gamut of emotions that ranged from eager anticipation to trembling fear, with most people simply registering a stoic acceptance of the fact.

Affiliation

It's not that we're sheep, getting pierced or cut just because everyone else is. I like to think it's because we're a very special group and we like doing something that sets us off from others. . . . You see all the guys at the bar and you know they are pierced and tattooed, and it gives you a good feeling to know you're one of them. . . . Happiness is standing in line at a cafeteria and detecting that the straight-looking babe in front of you has her nipples pierced. I don't really care what her sexual orientation is, I can relate to her.

Potential nonmainstream body modifiers frequently decide to alter their bodies because of a desire to identify themselves with a group of people they have deemed significantly important (for the importance of the tattoo as a mark of affiliation, see Sanders 1988b). Through the acquisition of a genital piercing or a brand for instance, individuals obtain a badge of admission—a visible record that affiliates them with others of similar interests and beliefs. Cross-culturally, clothing and hairstyles are the most obvious identifying mediums, and although important to the body modifiers in the study, neither carry the emotional wallop of the irreversible body mark. Whether one wishes to announce affiliation with the Hell's Angels, the Army or Navy, a youth gang, or any specific group, such body marks visually proclaim a sense of camaraderie to others so marked. Although affiliation with a desired group is typically a primary motivation for nonmainstream body modifiers, some individuals become involved because of the attendant disaffiliation from mainstream society. Similar to the tattooees in Sanders's (1988b) study, these individuals revel in the stigmatic power of their alterations. Genesis P-Orridge addressed this point in *Modern Primitives* (Vale and Juno 1989), noting

> I think if you're honest, there is also the enjoyment of being separated from the despicable *norm*. I remember giggling and feeling an amused, almost *smugness* going up the escalator after having the first Prince Albert piercing done. . . .I enjoyed that mysterious separation from the everyday. (p. 178)

Aesthetic

> God made my nipples beautiful, but my piercings made them even more so. . . . A brand on someone's thigh is very attractive, but so is any kind of mark that shows the person likes to play with his body. . . . My cutting is like a piece of fine art. . . . The brand I have now is on my back, but the next one I get will be on my arm so I can enjoy it all day.

The old adage "beauty is in the eye of the beholder" is particularly relevant to this motive, as the vast majority of people in the study regarded their alterations as well as those of others as an extraordinarily appealing addition to their bodies. As one devotee explained while examining the newly installed white gold circular barbell on her labia:

> Each time I get a piercing my boyfriend accuses me of gilding the lily, but I think my jewelry magically transforms a piece of flesh into a work of art.

Arnold Rubin, the editor of *Marks of Civilization* (1988), referred to body modification as "artistic transformation" and believed that the words "perfection" and "civilized" more accurately described the aesthetic quality and intentions of the phenomena than such popularly used negative terms as "deformation," "mutilation," and "disfigurement."

Whether the alteration was a piercing, branding, cutting, or burn mark, everyone involved in the process regarded the new decoration as a piece of art. Thus the recipients, the practitioners, and the audience graced the particular embellishment with such aesthetically descriptive words as gorgeous, elegant, lovely, magnificent, stunning, delicate, and exquisite.

Trust/Loyalty

> It meant a lot to me when Nathan fulfilled my wish that he get a Prince Albert.... Every slave I've had knew damn well he would have to prove his loyalty to me by getting pierced or branded. A good master would expect no less.... I was always afraid to get pierced because I knew it would hurt. But when Mistress told me it would reflect my trust and love for her, I did it.

Trust and loyalty was an especially important motive for the SM body modifiers in the study. Because SM play ranges from gentle to rough, with some scenes becoming potentially life threatening, there is constant talk about trust. No wonder, then, that the achievement of trust, and its companion, loyalty, are regarded by many SMers as the ultimate aphrodisiacs:

> SM is the anniversary when your lover has a gold ring put through your labia (and no anesthesia); then she holds you and says you're hers forever; and you'd do anything for her. (Miesen 1988, p. 37)

The irreversibility of a permanent body modification may be frightening to some people, but others find the prospects terribly appealing. Thus many couples, SM or non-SM, may regard piercing or a branding as a love token, at once a test and lasting symbol of trust and loyalty to each other. An interviewee expressed her feelings about the relationship between trust and her piercings this way:

> The whole thing boils down to who do you trust? Do you think I trust my supervisor not to fire me if he learned about this stuff? Come on! My life-style can only exist on trust. When I find myself in a promising relationship, a mutual piercing with some distinctive jewelry pumps up the trust level.

Religious/Mystic

> This body is my sacred vessel and I love to adorn it. . . . The overwhelming number of people I pierced or cut wanted it done for spiritual reasons. . . . I believe in archetypes. My labia piercings put me in touch with my early Egyptian sisters. . . . I like the way Fakir talks about mysticism and body play. That's why I have him do all my piercings. . . . Everything I do to my body is ritualistic.

It was not unusual to hear both the practitioners and the recipients of body alterations use religious/mystic reasons to account for their involvement in the process. Ganymede's description of his feelings about genital piercings is representative:

I know we are kin to those secret souls of so many cultures before. I know that this urge to pierce, to feel, to tattoo, to express with our very bodies in such primitive ways, is deep in the genetic memories, constant and strong as the tides. The chord it strikes resonates strongly for some of us, affecting our psyches, our spirits, our libidos. (Quoted in *PFIQ* no. 3, 1989, p. 31)

Fakir Musafer typically couches his "body play" activities in religious/mystic terms. Certainly, his flesh-skewering Sun Dance, his constant intertwining of permanent body alterations with talk of shamanic journeys, altered states, primal urges, Eastern religions, and so on serve as examples.

To many contemporary body modifiers, intentional body marks serve as a sacred chronicle to the individual's spiritual commitment. As Victor Turner (1987) aptly concluded,

It is clear that the body, whether clad or unclad, painted or unpainted, smooth or scarred, is never religiously neutral: it is always and everywhere a complex signifier of spirit, society, self and cosmos. (pp. 274–75)

Shock Value

I love it when they stare at me and their eyes scream "Deviant!" . . . Half the fun is walking down Powell with a big bone through my nose and watching those straight fuckers' jaws drop. . . . Frankly, the biggest kick for me is watching my friends' faces when I casually tell them my cock's got a ring through it. . . . Some of my so-called cool acquaintances try to look calm while we're talking, but I can tell they're blown away when I'm wearing my monster 4-gauge septum ring. I love it.

There were several opinions expressed regarding one's body modifications and the degree of shock they caused when viewed by others. No one professed that shock value was the primary motive for their involvement, but almost everyone had an observation or story about the reaction their alterations caused in one person or another.

Sanders (1988b) noted that tattooees gauged the reactions of strangers or casual associates in order to categorize them as compatible or noncompatible. Multiple piercers and branders use their body marks or piercings in a similar fashion.

Depending on the degree of association or the context of the encounter, some body modifiers were genuinely tickled when someone registered shock, whereas others were embarrassed. Among strangers, a few brandished their marks and accoutrements like a feisty porcupine, purposely inviting a gawk, leer, or odious comment. Yet in the company of friends or other body modifiers, someone with outlandish "jumbo jewelry" or a particularly salacious tattoo would garner admiring glances and appreciative comments.

Conclusions

Taken as a whole, the responses from my informants portray a group of individuals who for a variety of reasons enthusiastically involve themselves in nonmainstream body modification. They readily admit that their body modification interests are statistically outside the average range, but none transfer this conclusion to a statement regarding a deficiency in mental health. The medical literature on the topic presents a picture of deeply disturbed individuals engaging in self-mutilation for various psychopathological reasons (for an understanding of the medical interpretation of self-mutilation, see American Psychiatric Association 1987; Eckert 1977; Greilsheimer and Grover 1979; Pao 1969; Phillips and Muzaffer 1961; Tsunenari et al. 1981). This view is supported by the general nonparticipating public. My empirical observations lead me to disagree with the latter assessment. The overwhelming number of people in my study appear to be remarkably conventional sane individuals. Informed, educated, and employed in good jobs, they are functional and successful by social standards.

Given the motivations and rationale for body modification provided by the respondents, and their awareness of the ceremonial nature surrounding the bestowal and receiving of such nonmainstream alterations as branding, cutting, and genital piercing, it is possible to generate some conclusions regarding the phenomenon in contemporary United States. The worldwide practice of rites of passage, the rich body of ritual symbolism accompanying such rites, and the use of body ornamentation as a symbolic language provide the basis for such conclusions.

The individual and group dynamics of rites of passage in traditional non-Western cultures are strikingly similar to those I observed at body modification events in this study. In addition to Sanders's (1988b) recognition of the ritualized initiatory aspects of tattooing in America, Musafer argued that some people are instinctively driven to undergo a rite of passage to the point that they will invent one if society does not provide one. He also stipulated that such ritual must be painful, bloody, and mark producing. The recognition of a need for an initiatory experience is one reason why the term "modern primitive" is popular with many contemporary American body modifiers.

Affiliation is one of the most important functions of a rite of passage. The unknown, untested individual needs to be introduced to the known quantity—the social group. In his seminal work on ritual and symbols among the Ndembu, Victor Turner (1976) observed that the Ndembu visualize ritual symbols as "blazes" or "landmarks," "something that connects the unknown with the known" (p. 48). Turner also concluded:

> One aspect of the process of ritual symbolization among the Ndembu is, therefore, to make visible, audible, and tangible beliefs, ideas, values, sentiments, and psychological dispositions that cannot directly be perceived. (pp. 49–50)

The body modifiers in my study, like Ndembu initiates, have determined the importance of making visible, audible, and tangible what may have been previously unperceived. In Turner's reasoning, people getting a genital piercing would be using their bodies as symbolic conduits between their inner beings and the values, sentiments, and beliefs possessed by their desired social group. For the purpose of affiliation with a desired social order, people surrender what is dearest to every human being: the body itself. When viewed this way, modification of the surface of the body is more than a visible badge of admission; it is also a primary connector of one's psyche to one's social group.

Turner's belief that any complex or dominant symbol may stand for many things—"multivocality"—is also instructive in understanding why respondents in my study frequently provided several reasons for their involvement in body modification. For example, a clitoral piercing is a single dominant symbol, yet, as such, it carries with it a spectrum of referents—what Turner refers to as "significata." A young woman with a newly installed gold lock on her labia may express a multiplicity of significata ranging from sexual enhancement to chastity, from aesthetics to shock value. Thus we see how a single body modification may announce that its possessor is in harmony with an entire system of beliefs and values.

In a similar vein, Terrence Turner (1969) concluded that body decorations have like functions in all societies. In his studies of the Northern Kayapo of Brazil, Turner observed that such body ornamentations and modifications as lip plugs, earplugs, penis sheaths, and body painting express a symbolic language that reveals information regarding a person's social status, sex, and age. More profoundly, such body symbols "establish a channel of communication *within* the individual between the social and bio-logical aspects of his personality" (p. 105, emphasis in original).

Anthony Seeger's (1975) explanation of body ornamentation among the Suya of central Brazil has a firm base in the insights of both Victor Turner and Terrence Turner and confirms the impor-tant role that ritual symbolism plays in American nonmainstream body modification. Examining the human sensory faculties of hearing, speaking, and vision, Seeger sought to understand how the spectacular ornamentation of Suya ears and lips was related to the symbolic meaning that the society attached to each.

Seeger's observation that the body is "socialized" through such ornamentation agrees with the Victor Turner and Terrence Turner works cited above. In addition, Seeger's "organ importance" logic may be extended to the prominence that the body modifiers in my study placed on sexuality, as evidenced by their genital and nipple piercings. As surely as the Suya highlight the importance of hearing by wearing large wooden discs in their earlobes, so the genital piercers in contemporary American society celebrate their sexual potency by sporting a Prince Albert in the head of a penis or a silver heart on a labia piercing.

The number of contemporary Americans who have become involved with nonmainstream body modification is presently small. However, it is important to remember that the practices discussed in this article are a relatively new phenomenon in this culture. Each year, American society is bombarded with new body alterations, many of which are quickly assessed as unacceptable for one reason or another and fail to enter mainstream society. However, recent history also shows that some initially rejected alterations may take hold in a subculture and eventually catapult their way into the larger society. For example, ear piercing in America moved from nonmainstream to mainstream society in less than a decade and multiple ear piercing among both males and females is now relatively common. Lip and nose piercing is increasingly tolerated, but whether nipple piercing will follow suit remains to be seen.

A growing number of people in American culture believe that the penis and the clitoris are just as deserving of gilding as are earlobes. These individuals, like the style setters in earlier times who defied American society's strictures on body alteration by experimenting with such daring embellishments as lipstick, rouge, painted nails, eye makeup, and radical hairstyles, join human beings around the world in using their bodies to express a symbolic language that reveals their sentiments, dispositions, and desired alliances. Through adornment, the naked skin moves one from the biological world to the cultural world. As David Levi-Strauss observed in Vale and Juno's (1989) book,

The unmarked body is a raw, inarticulate, mute body. It is only when the body acquires the "Marks of Civilization" that it begins to communicate and becomes an active part of the social body.

Notes

1. Of course, most so-called "irreversible" body modifications are not truly so. Tattoos fade, scars may flatten, cutting may heal without scars, and piercings, if not tended, will close.

2. A *Newsweek* magazine article (January 7, 1991) recognized the current popularity of tattooing in the United States and noted, "It's the most painful trend since whalebone corsets: tattooing, the art of the primitive and the outlaw, has been moving steadily into the fashion mainstream." This same article also observed that in the past twenty years, the number of professional tattoo studios had jumped from 300 to 4,000.

3. With the exception of the professional body modifiers highlighted in this article (e.g., Jim Ward, Fakir Musafer, Raelynn Gallina, and others), all names of individuals are fictitious.

4. Interestingly, today many tattooed people regard piercing, branding, and scarification as repugnant. For example, the following warning was displayed prominently on the wall of a Northern California tattoo studio (it was apparently part of a registration form for a 1982 national tattoo convention):

> This convention is for Tattoo Artists and Fans who care about the Tattoo Profession. Anyone breaking the following rules will be asked to leave with no refunds. Facial tattoos other than cosmetic (eyebrows, lines, etc.) not permitted. Piercing of the private parts of the anatomy not permitted to be shown at any time. Any facial piercing with bones, chains, etc. must be removed during entire convention.

5. I was accompanied at each workshop by Craig Moro, a Berkeley resident who had served several months as a volunteer for the San Francisco Sexual Information Switchboard (SIS), a call-in telephone service for people seeking sexual information.

6. The first occasion was a workshop on play piercing, a procedure that involves brief piercing with hypodermic or sewing needles, fishhooks, staples, and the like for fun and enjoyment and, unlike "permanent" piercing, is not done with the intention of installing some type of jewelry in the hole. After a lengthy introduction to the techniques, hygiene, and materials involved, the workshop leader divided audience volunteers into piercers and piercees. As a piercer, I selected an experienced partner to pierce, donned my rubber gloves, popped a hypodermic needle from its protective capsule using the recommended technique, and was within inches of making the jab when it suddenly occurred to me that I had some serious doubts about what I was doing. Even though the teacher was exquisitely clear on the need for care and safety during the "scene," my congenital clumsiness and concern about the blood being splattered here and there caused me to back out as gracefully as possible at that late instant. Another volunteer happily replaced me, and I don't believe my rapport was damaged by the event.

The second participation occurred during the workshop on playing with fire. Here it was simply a matter of overcoming my innate fear of being burned and joining the group of eager volunteers brushing each other with a lighted small torch soaked in a 70 percent solution of isopropyl alcohol. To my surprise, the activity was enjoyable and caused some of my fellow volunteers to wonder if I was considering changing my sexual proclivities.

7. The intellect of many SMers who I interviewed and observed during my fieldwork was confirmed to me at one San Francisco workshop entitled "Playing with Fire." During the workshop, the instructor's knowledgeable discourse on the ignition points of various isopropyl alcohols was interrupted by several audience members who had extemporaneously launched into an animated conversation on such matters as flammability versus combustionability, chemical structures of alcohol and gasoline, and the medical definitions and implications of the various types of skin burns. After listening to the display a few moments, the instructor broke in by expressing her astonishment at the esoteric outpouring, only to be sharply reminded by one audience member, "There are no dumb SMers!"

8. Because SM practices are so varied, it is difficult to provide a satisfactory single definition of SM behavior. Charles Moser, a psychotherapist who specializes in SM clients and wrote his Ph.D. dissertation on sadomasochism, uses five criteria to identify people involved in SM (in Truscott 1989): (1) appearance of dominance and submission,

(2) role-playing, (3) consensuality, (4) sexual content, and (5) mutual definition (i.e., people involved recognize that what they are doing is different from the "norm"). Townsend (1983) suggested "a short list of characteristics" that he believed are present in most scenes that he would classify as SM: a dominant-submissive relationship, a giving and receiving of pain that is pleasurable to both parties, fantasy and role-playing, humiliation, fetish involvement, and the acting out of one or more ritualized interactions (bondage, flagellation, etc.).

SM does not have to involve pain. There are many people who prefer a gentler approach to what otherwise would be considered SM; thus one sees the letters "D and S" for "dominance and submission," or "B and D" for "bondage and discipline." For an extended discussion of the pain issue, see Baumeister (1988), Gebhard (1969), Reik (1957), and Weinberg (1987).

For a scholarly presentation of SM behavior, see Weinberg's (1987) review of recent sociological literature on sadomasochism in the United States. For a nonacademic but informative introduction to SM behavior, I recommend two popular books by insiders: *Urban Aboriginals* (Mains 1984) and *The Leatherman's Handbook 2* (Townsend 1983). Because these sources are male-oriented (very little academic work has appeared regarding female SM), the reader interested in female SM will find helpful the *Sandmutopia Guardian and Dungeon Journal or Dungeonmaster* magazine. Pat Califia has also written knowledgeably of the lesbian SM community (see Califia 1987).

Not surprising, the SM people I interviewed were infuriated with the standard psychological characterization of SM as aberrant behavior. For example, the *DSM–III–R*, the official diagnostic manual for the American Psychiatric Association, lists both sadism and masochism as psychosexual disorders.

9. Other Powerhouse workshops scheduled during my fieldwork period were Creative Bondage, Electrical Toys, Clothespins and Staples, Male Tit and Genitorture, Tit Play, Cock and Ball Torture, Whipping and Caning, Mummification, and Equestrian Restraints.

10. The church's liberal reputation was confirmed to me one sunny Saturday afternoon as our group huddled over a spread-legged woman undergoing a clitoris hood piercing to the accompaniment of an a cappella choir rehearsing Handel's "Hallelujah Chorus" in a downstairs room—a surrealistic scene that would not have escaped Van Gennep.

11. It as not unusual to hear SM people remark on whether a par-

ticular body modification or play technique would produce a genital orgasm or an equal thrill in the mind ("head orgasm") or both.

12. A distinction may be made between two different types of burning that I witnessed during my fieldwork with the SM body modifiers. One type, as described in the Musafer burning demonstration, was intended to leave a mark. Another type, "play burning," capitalizes on the classic SM goals of trust and the threat of pain and/or injury, but does so without leaving intentional burn marks. The ritual use of fire in SM scenes is not uncommon. The cross-cultural use of fire as a means of "cooking" a person symbolically was discussed by Levi-Strauss (1970). See also Tonkinson (1978) on the use of fire on Mardudjara initiates and Warner (1964) on fire jumping among the Ngoni.

13. It is this penchant for scholarly analysis, and concomitant diversity of conclusions that caused J. E. Cawte (1973) to describe the phenomenon of subincision (penis slitting, or "whistlecock") among certain Australian aborigines as "complexly overdetermined" (p. 390).

14. Of course, some individuals fell into more than one category. The quoted statements in each category were selected to represent typical responses for that category. Ellipses (. . .) indicate a separate response from a different informant.

References

American Psychiatric Association. 1987. *Diagnostic and Statistical Manual of Mental Disorders*, 3d ed. Washington, D.C.: American Psychiatric Association.

Baumeister, R. 1988. "Masochism as Escape from Self." *Journal of Sex Research* 25: 29.

Bilmes, J., and A. Howard. 1980. "Pain as Cultural Drama." *Anthropology and Humanism Quarterly* 5: 10–12.

Brain, D. 1979. *The Decorated Body*. New York: Harper & Row.

Brown, J. 1963. "A Cross-cultural Study of Female Initiation Rites." *American Anthropologist* 65: 837–53.

Califia, P. 1987. "A Personal View of the History of the Lesbian Community and Movement in San Francisco," in *Samois: Coming to Power*, pp. 243–87. Boston: Alyson.

Cawte, J. 1973. "Why We Slit the Penis," in *The Psychology of Aboriginal Australians*, ed. G. E. Kearney, P. R. deLacy, and G. R. Davidson, p. 390. New York: Wiley.

Ebin, V. 1979. *The Body Decorated*. London: Thames & Hudson.

Eckert, G. 1977. "The Pathology of Self-mutilation and Destructive Acts: A Forensic Study and Review." *Journal of Forensic Sciences* 22: 54.

Gebhard, P. 1969. "Fetishism and Sadomasochism," in *Dynamics of Deviant Sexuality*, ed. J. H. Masserman, pp. 71–80. New York: Grune & Stratton.

Gould, R. 1968. "Masculinity and Mutilation in a Primitive Society." *Medical Opinion and Review* 4: 59–75.

Gollwitzer, P. 1986. "Striving for Specific Identities: The Social Reality of Self-symbolizing," in *Public Self and Private Self*, ed. R. Baumeister, pp. 143–59. New York: Springer Verlag.

Govenar, A. 1977. "The Acquisition of Tattooing Competence: An Introduction." *Folklore Annual of the University Folklore Association* 7 and 8.

Greilsheimer, H., and J. Grover. 1979. "Male Genital Self-mutilation." *Archives of General Psychiatry* 36: 441 .

Levi-Strauss, C. 1970. *The Raw and the Cooked*. New York: Harper.

Mains, G. 1984. *Urban Aboriginals*. San Francisco: Gay Sunshine Press.

Miesen, D. 1988. "SM: A View of Sadomasochism." *Sandmutopia Guardian and Dungeon Journal* 3: 37.

Nichols, M. 1985. "The Piercing Profile Evaluated." *Piercing Fans International Quarterly* 24: 14–15.

Pao, P. 1969. "The Syndrome of Delicate Self-cutting." *British Journal of Medical Psychiatry* 42: 195.

Phillips, R., and A. Muzaffer. 1961. "Aspects of Self-mutilation in the Population of a Large Psychiatric Hospital." *Psychiatric Quarterly* 35: 421.

Reik, T. 1957. *Masochism in Modern Man*. New York: Grove.

Rubin, A. 1988. *Marks of Civilization*. Los Angeles: Museum of Cultural History.

Sanders, C. 1986. "Tattooing as Fine Art and Client Work: The Art Work of Carl (Shotsie) Gorman." *Appearances* 12: 12–13.

———. 1988a. "Drill and Fill: Client Choice, Client Typologies and Interactional Control in Commercial Tattoo Settings," in *Marks of Civilization*, ed. A. Rubin, pp. 219–31. Los Angeles: Museum of Cultural History.

———. 1988b. "Marks of Mischief: Becoming and Being Tattooed." *Journal of Contemporary Ethnography* 16: 395–432.

———. 1989. *Customizing the Body: The Art and Culture of Tattooing*. Philadelphia: Temple University Press.

Seeger, A. 1975. "The Meaning of Body Ornaments: A Suya Example." *Ethnology* 14: 211–23.

St. Clair, L., and A. Govenar. 1981. *Stoney Knows How: Life as a Tattoo Artist.* Lexington: University Press of Kentucky.

Thevos, M. 1984. *The Painted Body.* New York: Rizzoli.

Tonkinson, R. 1978. *The Mardudjara Aborigines: Living the Dream in Australia's Desert.* New York: Holt, Rinehart & Winston.

Townsend, L. 1983. *The Leatherman's Handbook 2.* New York: Modernismo.

Trigger, B. 1969. *The Huron: Farmers of the North.* New York: Holt, Rinehart & Winston.

Truscott, C. 1989. "Interview with a Sexologist: Dr. Charles Moser." *Sandmutopia Guardian and Dungeon Journal* 4: 23–24.

Tsunenari, S., et al. 1981. "Self-mutilation: Plastic Spherules in Penile Skin in Yakuza, Japan's Racketeers." *American Journal of Forensic Medical Pathology* 2: 203.

Turner, T. 1969. "Cosmetics: The Language of Bodily Adornment," in *Conformity and Conflict: Readings in Cultural Anthropology,* 5th ed., ed. J. Spradley and D. McCurdy, pp. 98–107. Boston: Little, Brown.

Turner, V. 1976. *The Forest of Symbols: Aspects of Ndembu Ritual.* Ithaca, N.Y.: Cornell University Press.

———. 1987. "Bodily Marks," in *Encyclopedia of Religion,* ed. M. Eliade, 2: 274–75. New York: Macmillan.

Vale, V., and A. Juno. 1989. *Modern Primitives.* San Francisco: Re/Search.

Van Gennep, A. 1960. *The Rites of Passage.* Chicago: University of Chicago Press.

Warner, W. L. 1964. *A Black Civilization: A Study of an Australian Tribe.* New York: Harper.

Weinberg, T. 1987. "Sadomasochism in the United States: A Review of Recent Sociological Literature." *Journal of Sex Research* 23: 50–69.

Wicklund, R., and P. Gollwitzer. 1982. *Symbolic Self-completion.* Hillsdale, N.J.: Lawrence Erlbaum.

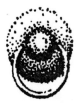

Of the exotic piercing done today the most popular and common is **nipple** piercing. It seems strange that something this popular has virtually no traceable, historical precedent. There are passing references to its having been done by society women during the reigns of Louis XIV and Queen Victoria to enhance the size and shape of the nipples. It is said to have been practiced by the Kabyle, a Berber tribe of northern Algeria, and some unidentified Native American tribe from what is now Texas.

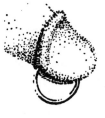

Navel piercings were worn by ancient Egyptian royalty and denied to commoners. Today the piercing is one of the most popular. Exotic dancers love it because it is very eye-catching especially when adorned with a flashing jewel.

Of the male genital piercings, the most common and sensuous is the **Prince Albert**, also called a Dressing Ring by Victorian haberdashers. Its purpose was allegedly to strap the penis tight against the leg, thus minimizing any "unsightly" bulge in the extremely tight trousers popular at the time. Supposedly Prince Albert had such a piercing which served the additional purpose of keeping the foreskin retracted and thus keeping his member sweet-smelling so as not to offend the queen. Today the piercing is almost exclusively for erotic stimulation.

The second most popular penis piercing is that of the **frenum** (or frenulum). The name is anatomical. The piercing itself goes side-to-side through the loose flesh on the underside of the penis between a quarter and a half inch behind the Prince Albert. This makes it possible for men to have both piercings, and many men do.

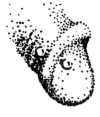

Dydoe piercing is usually done in pairs through the glans penis at the three and nine o'clock positions when the penis is viewed head-on. Short Barbell Studs usually about 3/8" long, are the jewelry of choice.

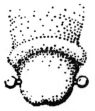

The **ampallang** is the best and most extensively documented of all exotic body piercings. Mentioned in the logs of many explorers and condemned by missionaries, it is found in Borneo, New Guinea, and some parts of the Philippines. The piercing is horizontal through the head of the penis usually above the urethra, although authorities disagree on this point. Its primary function is to stimulate the female during intercourse.

As described in the Kama Sutra, the ancient classic Hindu treatise on love and social conduct, the **apadravya** is any one of a number of devices (antique "French Ticklers" and/or dildoes, if you will) used during intercourse to excite the woman. Among the Dravidian people of southern India, the word also refers to the device worn in a vertical piercing through the head of a man's penis.

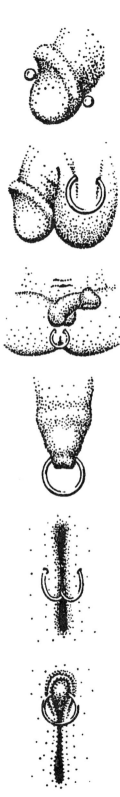

In some Arabic cultures the scrotums of boys are pierced when they reach puberty. The piercing was said to be done as a rite of passage and was called a **hafada**. It was placed high on the side of the scrotum near the base of the penis.

The **guiche** (pronounced "geesh") is said to be indigenous to the South Pacific, primarily Tahiti. Placement of the piercing is through the *raphe perinei*, the ridge of skin between the scrotum and the anus, at a point corresponding roughly with the inseam of a pair of pants. Once the piercing heals bangles can be attached.

While genital piercings are primarily done for erotic stimulation, they have been done in certain times and places to prohibit sexual indulgence. In ancient Greece and Rome this was commonly done to male slaves by piercing their **fore-skins** and inserting a locking device called a *fibula*. The practice was called *infibulation*.

Women, too, have been infibulated. This was done in many locales—Ethiopia, Rome, India, and Persia, to name a few—by piercing the **labia** lips and inserting some kind of locking device. The purpose was to assure that the woman didn't dally with a man other than her husband, or, in the case of slaves, a man not approved by her owner.

Clitoris piercings are among the rarest one is ever likely to encounter. The primary reason is that most women don't possess a clit large enough to pierce.

Piercing illustrations and text courtesy of
Gauntlet, Inc., San Francisco, CA.

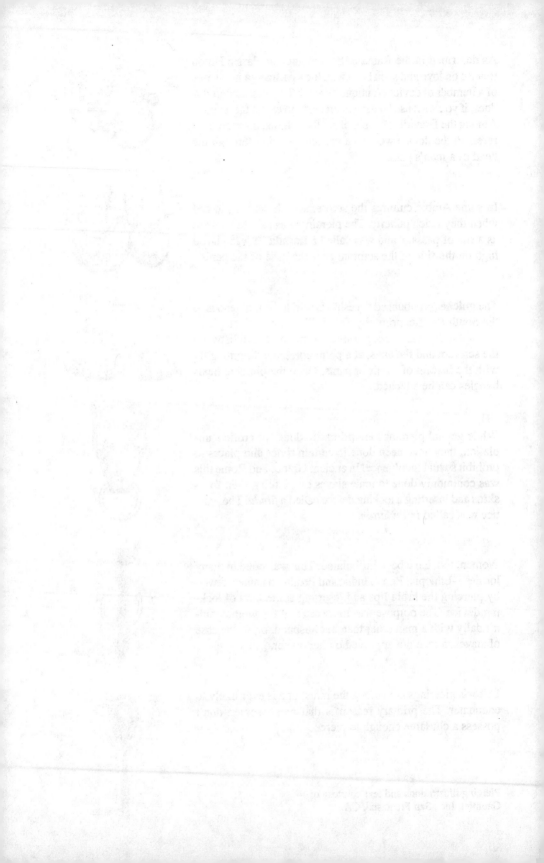

Joel I. Brodsky

The Mineshaft:
A Retrospective Ethnography

The Mineshaft was a bar and sex club which operated for a number of years in New York's meat-packing district on the lower West Side of Manhattan. This bar gained great notoriety among gay men, was discussed in the gay press, and used as the setting for pornographic stories. Late in 1985, in an atmosphere of lurid headlines, right-wing agitation, and panic over AIDS in the public school system, it was closed by order of New York State authorities for clearly political reasons (see Rist 1985). In what follows I try to describe the Mineshaft in such a way as to ground it in sociological and anthropological theory.

Specifically, I present an overall ethnography of the Mineshaft in cultural and institutional context. My aim is to suggest some answers to the question, "What did going to the Mineshaft do for those who went there?" While it is obvious, if not tautological, that customers in a sex club ordinarily obtain or hope to obtain sexual gratification by their participation, the question arises why in one such place and not another? Indeed, why in a

© 1993 Haworth Press, Binghamton, New York. *Journal of Homosexuality* 24 (3/4): 233–51.

sex club, as opposed to the privacy and intimacy of a monogamous relationship at home? And if in a sex club, why in ways
quite so contradictory of dominant cultural standards (as were
some common Mineshaft practices such as handballing, micturi-
tion, and S&M)? My contention is that the Mineshaft performed
a variety of integrative social and cultural functions for gay men
at the communal level, and that these functions were manifest in
its physical and social structure and setting.

My analysis begins with a brief review of the literature on
male recreational S&M which I believe offers a key to understanding the Mineshaft's cultural base. Then, after a brief note
on my methodology and limitations, I present my retrospective
data and findings.

Male Recreational S&M:
Fetish and Fantasy in America

The Mineshaft was, by reputation, an "S&M" bar, and a well-
known site to gay men of the late 1970s whom Mains (1984) would
have described as "leathermen." Its customers evinced a hypermasculine style of dress and an ethos which posited sexual excitement as a self-justified basis for meaningful human relationships.
In contrast to the dominant culture's requirement that eroticism be
linked to gender relations, and thus that "real men" only desire
women, the Mineshaft articulated the principle that "real men" not
only can and do desire other "real men," but that "real men" can
be *exclusively* homosexual. In order to examine this relationship
between a gay male "S&M" bar and changes in the gender system,
it is important to clarify what "S&M" means to gay men.

In the 1970s gay men found themselves strongly at odds
with the dominant system of erotic norms. While the dominant
system continued to be heterosexist, rationalized, materialist,
power-oriented, and erotophobic, a counterculture prevailed
among gay men which was in many respects Dionysian (see
Maffesoli 1983). So, for example, while both these systems could

have been described as "phallocentric," phalli themselves remained invisible, kept secret and taboo in the imagery of the dominant system; while the counterculture, itself denied visibility, encouraged playfulness with and admiration of phalli. It has been claimed that a majority of American males experience homoerotic arousal, and perhaps half experience orgasm while engaged in homosexual behavior at some point in their lives. Yet male homoeroticism in the United States is legitimated with only extreme difficulty, and most men try to forget their pubescent sexual experimentation.

A significant contrast with many precapitalist societies concerns societal norms for rites of passage into adult male roles. Rather than being normatively initiated into a male *communitas* (see Turner 1969), American males are normatively inducted into patriarchal, heterosocial bureaucratic structures. In fact, there is a dearth of universalized sacred rites of passage in American society. All of these characteristics can be viewed (e.g., by some gay men) as alienating and oppressive defects in the American system. My argument is that the Mineshaft functioned for some participants to address these defects, with partial success. Insofar as it did succeed, it took on meaning within the gay male community as a place of transformative experience and possibly awesome rituals.

"S&M" can be interpreted as "sadomasochism" or "Slave/ Master" (Townsend 1983, pp. 14–17). The latter meaning suggests two aspects of S&M: (1) Since slavery was abolished in the United States in 1863 it is not surprising that researchers have discovered that S&M is a kind of playacting or game; and (2) though a game, it is concerned with some of the more profound sociocultural contradictions in American culture.[1] Responding to the first meaning ("sadism" and "masochism," as per Krafft-Ebing 1965) the literature discusses "recreational S&M," which it sharply distinguishes from popular and medicalized usages of "sadistic" and "masochistic" to refer to, respectively, cruel brutality and pathological self-destructiveness. Masochism of the latter sort is common among oppressed people in the form of "guilt-expiation rituals," and is often manifested among gay men appearing before psychiatrists (Adam 1978, p. 101), for whom psychiatric treatment is such a ritual. Empirical sociological studies of male recreational S&M (see Spengler 1983/1977) have been rare and hermeneutic, but are more than adequate to discredit Krafft-Ebing's pathologizing concept of an inevitable progression of disease from "atavistic manifestations" to "the most monstrous acts of destruction." S&M is posited as a "career" which some gay men will follow and which begins with an early disenchantment with the gay world (Kamel 1983a, p. 75). It is critical for initiates firstly to come to view "leathersex" as a process in which psychosexual fulfillment is mutual and can only be achieved interdependently, and secondly to develop their acting skills (ibid., p. 77). For this reason, supposedly, novices prefer submissive roles in which the script is seemingly prescribed. At some later point the initiate is likely to become a dominant partner himself (ibid.). Catalogs of paraphiliac activities which constitute the discursive universe of S&M have also been elaborated (Kamel 1983a; Weinberg 1983/1978) and include: pain, bondage, humiliation, domination, and watersports. Featured are analyses of dyadic relationships such as "master/slave." In Kamel's (1983b) scenario leathersex uses restraint (either physical or psychological) to establish dyadic roles, humiliation to carry them out, and fear to maintain them. Prior to erotic interaction participants use costume to signal desires to prospective partners and often verbally negotiate the question "what-do-you-like-to-do?" Frequently S&M sexual activity "culminates in masculine gentleness, warmth, and affection" (ibid., p. 171).

The final stage described by Kamel (1983a) in the development of the S&M career is a stage he calls "limiting," a period of deliberate experimentation with activities during which the experimenter establishes the boundaries of "his S&M tastes." This concept points directly to Lee's notion of socially organized risk reduction (discussed below), and Kamel claims that many of the implicit rules of the leather world revolve around this notion of limits. For example, a sadist's reputation hinges on his ability to decode and abide by a partner's limits. Individuals experimenting with "limiting" would clearly benefit from an environment where liminality, in the sense of threshold experience, particularly sensory threshold experience, could be engaged in while experienced persons willing and able to assist were present. It will be clear that the Mineshaft provided such an environment.[2]

At the community level, Lee (1983) and Weinberg (1983/1978) are concerned with the sociology of risk. They argue that sadomasochism is theater, invoking Goffman's concept of the "theatrical frame." What ideally occurs in the S&M world, says Weinberg (1983, p. 106) quoting Goffman, is that participants "play the world backwards" and "the individual can arrange to script what is to come, unwinding his own reel." Through appropriate social organization the S&M world functions to reduce actual risks. Dyads and sex clubs are viewed as desirable means of creating and maintaining social support networks among participants.

Murray (1984, p. 42) points out that the theatrical realization of fantasy and the reality of behavioral risk-taking may often coincide in S&M, and that not all participants in S&M scenes may "maintain role distance" well as "adepts." Yet he agrees that S&M is theater, and argues on this basis, that the emergence of S&M in the 1970s may be part of a transition "from Mother Camp to Father Camp." In this respect he sees "a continuity between female and male drag in the common focus on costuming and in choreographing near-caricatures of gender."

But who is the audience for this theater? Is it the hostile, oppressive heterosexual world, or is it the gay world itself? And Murray's own question remains unanswered: Why does this shift emerge at this particular time in this particular way?

Goffman argues (1963) the possibility of a minority within a minority being created, a community of deviants within a deviant community. The "shift" Murray describes is an emergence into *gay* discourse of an S&M controversy. It occurs about the time the Mineshaft opened in the mid-70s. At this time, in response to the new aspirations and conditions of greater tolerance created by the Gay Liberation movement, the traditionally closed S&M world was becoming more open and accessible to "non-adept" gay men. As it did so, the hypermasculine S&M style of dress and eroticism increasingly challenged the stereotypical equation of open gay identity and gender reversal (see Newton 1972, p. 24). S&M styles became at least a widely understood means of signaling desire for other men. But this change also brought to light an elaborate subculture available to gay men which systematically violated taboos against a wide range of sexual behaviors in addition to those against male homosexual relations. This was a time when gay bars were beginning to drop their traditional practices of hiding in remote locations behind blacked out windows, and becoming more visible. In this context of increasingly conceivable legitimacy for some as yet undefined gay male role in American society the new style appeared to some as a politically liable display of dirty linen. Indeed, if the Mineshaft exaggeratedly caricatured anything, it was a camp version of the gay past.[3]

If the Mineshaft is to be understood as an embodiment of "Father Camp," then the process by which "camp" itself becomes meaningful must be sought within the gay male world. I would suggest that camp has an interior, deadly serious side: perhaps an unnamed side associated with the neglected socialization needs of gay men.[4] The serious side of "Father Camp" might be the lack of institutionalized anticipatory socialization for male erotic relationships in American society. Behind S&M as theater might be a genuine compensation for this lack.

Murray also criticizes the view that S&M emerges more distinctly with diversification of the gay community, as implying that there is a "reservoir" of repressed S&M eroticism waiting to fill the expanding capacity. In effect, his criticism is that this is an essentialist argument.

Yet, as even Krafft-Ebing acknowledges, there may be a physiological basis for S&M which is inherent and normal in human sexual response. It seems to be the case cross-culturally that any adrenal arousal brings human beings physiologically closer to sexual arousal. If so, the view that S&M emerges more distinctly with diversification of the gay community is not an essentialist claim, but emphasizes the role of culture in shaping and differentiating erotic from violent behavior. It emphasizes the cultural distinctiveness of patterns of life in the gay world: a sociocultural world which has, in dramatic contrast to the hegemonic "Rambo" culture of the contemporary United States, preferred the eroticization of adrenalin to the adrenalization of eros.

Method

What follows is retrospectively based on numerous observations and conversations in the Mineshaft between the spring of 1979 and winter of 1982, and recent conversations with a small number of friends who also observed the Mineshaft. All of these observations were made from the perspective of participants in the role of customers, rather than employees or managers of the Mineshaft. The Mineshaft was, however, a consumer-oriented business which functioned in a capitalist social context. These observations thus reflect an experiential impression that was "managed" with the intent of attracting and pleasing customers. The observations extend to a variety of customer subroles, including nonclub member and club member; weekday night "regular," and weekend night "tourist" and "novice" or "initiate." In short, some observations were made on weekends, during periods of employment in the "straight" world; while others were made during periods of unemployment when the Mineshaft served as an important communal focus for the researcher.

The observations are retrospective, and may suffer from the fallibility of memory, as opposed to systematic observation: they are selective, and are certainly not representative or random. As an ethnography, this study is rather incomplete. Since the data do not exist, I do not attempt to analyze the details of interaction in the Mineshaft; the glances, gestures, movements, and language(s). Since the site is closed, more systematic research and analysis will not be possible.

The Institutional Context of a Commercial Anti-Structure

The Mineshaft operated in a highly developed market economy which provided services to gay men.[5] It began operation as an "after-hours" "leather" bar in the "Triangle" district, three terms whose explanation below will clarify the bar's market position. But more than a service, the Mineshaft was a focal point for symbolic ritual activity among gay men, and itself eventually acquired symbolic and political/media significance. For example, the movie *Cruising* began shooting on location in several S&M bars in New York, and a version of the interior of the Mineshaft was featured prominently in one vivid scene. While permission to shoot the movie had been granted the director, Stanley Freidkin, by various bar owners, the expectations that were raised in the gay male community that a "quality" movie would feature their lifestyle turned to rage when the nature of the script became known. This script recreated several actual sex-related Greenwich Village murders of gay men and implied that such violence was inherent in the world of leather and S&M, and indeed, in gay community life (Russo 1981, p. 236). Such distortions implicitly legitimated antigay violence as beyond the control of rational political authority (while the actual murders remained unsolved). The gay male community's anti-*Cruising* rage produced in 1979 the most severe gay/police confrontations in New York between the Stonewall riots of 1969 and the Liberty Centennial riots of 1986. (The latter protested the Burger court's antigay decision in the *Hardwick* v *Georgia* case.) It did not, however, prevent *Cruising*'s dissemination of exploitative and homophobic images of gay male life, in the established Hollywood tradition (see Russo 1981).

Given Friedkin's history as the director of the much despised

Boys in the Band, the trust exhibited by the bar owners in retrospect seems naive at best. But Russo notes (ibid., p. 233) that gay men working in the film wrote an article at the time in the popular magazine *Mandate* explaining that their participation in the film was intended to project a new, masculine, gay image to the American public. In other words, some gay men perceived the Mineshaft and its world as symbolic manifestations of their own carefully constructed masculinity. Some believed that a deeply homophobic culture would attribute the same positive meaning to the Mineshaft that these actors did. Perhaps the community's rage would more appropriately have been directed at the culture that rejected their lifestyle than at the film's portrayal of it. It is clear, in any case, that from the perspective of that dominant culture, the Mineshaft was a convenient, hazily perceived, confirmation of homophobic stereotypes of sexual evil and violence.

The "triangle" was a small triangular-shaped block formed by an odd intersection in Manhattan's meat-packing district along the Hudson River just north of the West Village, and just southwest of the Chelsea district. Few lived in the triangle district, and the city's repeated efforts to run a major expressway through it lowered its commercial value, as meat-packing plants nervously sought to relocate just across the river in New Jersey. At night this anomalous urban landscape of nineteenth-century meat-packing plants with their covered sidewalks was silent and deserted. At the same time it was geographically convenient to a variety of gay districts. It proved an ideal location for a series of after-hours clubs and bars devoted to sexual/legal marginality. For example, the "Anvil" featured a large stage where those not engaging in other sexual or social activity could watch paid performers engage in extraordinary feats, on occasion with members of the audience.

It is likely that the floorshow at the Anvil popularized previously limited sexual practices such as "fisting," or handballing. During the period of observation informants made recurrent references to a legendary performance at the Anvil during which an adult female member of a family prominent in national politics allegedly got up from the audience and "fisted" an onstage performer. As this story implies, the Anvil (and the Mineshaft) had pretensions to attract members of the American elite. Whether this was at all the case, is not clear, but both bars often had long lines to get in, not a few limousines at their entrances, and long lines of taxis outside when people were leaving. Other bars in the triangle were less glamorous. The Mineshaft did not feature staged performances so much as a large space and multifunctional facilities for a full complement of sexual activities which ranged from "vanilla" sex to fisting, whipping, and the use of hot candle wax.

"After-hours" bars were bars that operated after the legal closing hours of the "regular" bars. They began to proliferate in the early 1970s, benefitting from a hands-off political attitude that characterized municipal government at that time (probably maintained through graft) and from the relative safety they offered to those who had been for many years engaging in so-called anonymous sexual encounters in a variety of increasingly dangerous open-air sites in Greenwich Village along or close to the Hudson River. They survived the test of a raid by federal agents of nine such bars on the evening of July 17, 1971 (Weinberg and Williams 1974, pp. 40–41). So, too, did the Mafia links that the raid was ostensibly intended to thwart. During the period of observation the Mineshaft itself was closed down for several weeks of the busy winter season. One rumor suggested that this was because of its lack of a liquor license. Another said that the Gay Men's Health Crisis, a community group, had discovered amoebas, the protozoans responsible for amebiasis, growing on the walls. At any event, it was much cleaner when it reopened and smelled less fetid.

Different after-hours bars attracted different crowds, had different entrance requirements, and featured different atmospheres and activities. A common feature of after-hours bars was their "backroom" function, that is the sheltering of sexual activity. After the "regular" bars closed, their remaining patrons would migrate to the after-hours bars where they could be assured of sexual activity.[6] Employees of the regular bars would also go to the after-hours bars to relax after work. These bars were thus complementary in their market functioning to the regular bars, encouraging customers to stay until closing and reducing social pressures to meet and arrange sexual encounters. At the same time they competed for customers with other late-night or all-night establishments which sheltered sexual activity such as the bath-houses and discos. In competing with the bath-houses and discos they generally offered lower admission costs and the availability of alcoholic beverages. The Mineshaft, in the rather thin guise of being a "private club," provided alcoholic beverages to patrons in exchange for "donations," and the $5.00 admission for a nonmember would include use of the coat-check room and a "free" beer. Bathhouses and discos cost more, forbade alcohol, and offered greater prestige as places to go in some gay circles.

"Leather" bars were foci for the S&M world, and I have suggested that this world intersected the gay male world in such a way as to provide a measure of "in-group deviance" (Goffman 1963, p. 145) in relation to the latter. The S&M world has its own institutions, which include: dyads and social networks, specialty bars and clubs (which may or may not be "after hours"), publications, political organizations, and motorcycle clubs. Kamel (1983b) describes the cultural outlook of "leathermen" as distinct from both heterosexual S&M participants and other gay men who have not developed an "S&M career." Kamel claims that "leathermen" are devoted to "the ultimate in man-to-man interaction." That gay male S&M is not universally so perceived among gay men is fairly obvious. In the traditional "Mother Camp" slang among gay men in the ghetto, the term "leather queen," not "leatherman" was used. Such usage included a complex set of pejorative meanings: (1) There is an implication that S&M is a sexual specialty or fetish like any other and available to any gay man so inclined, since the formula noun + queen (Dynes 1985, p. 119) implies an extreme of sexual specialization; e.g., "I thought he was just an ordinary queen, I didn't know he was a leather queen." (2) There is an implication that S&Mers' claims to ultramasculinity and more meaningful sexual experience are suspect, since the term "queen" has semantic roots which imply an "impudent woman, jade, or hussy" (ibid.). In a variant usage, leathermen were referred to as "leather girls," a word play on the British movie *The Leather Boys*, which is about the unrequited love of a gay male biker for a heterosexual biker. The pejorative connotations of these usages could have expressed a wish among many gay men to distinguish themselves categorically from S&M gay men, to cognitively bound gay S&M, and may have disguised a latent fear and insecurity about S&M. Or, on the contrary, as Stephen Murray suggests (personal communication), shown a familiarity-bred contempt for and skepticism of the leathermen's own distancing. At any rate, in spite of the ideological boundary between the leather and nonleather worlds, it is clear that "leathermen" and "normal gays" were highly interdependent components of the gay male ghetto. From the literature one would expect that the S&M world received a sizeable complement of initiates from the gay world at large. Indeed, in comparatively observing crowds in S&M and "normal" gay bars, one would be struck by the relatively larger proportion of older men in the former.

Inside the Mineshaft:
Layout, Rules, Stages, Props, Acts

The Mineshaft could be approached with a sense of abandon, reverence, anxious dread (typically the first time), but usually evoked some sense of excitement, however mild. On weekends few arrived before 2:00 A.M. and the crowd was dense until at least 5:00 A.M., but on weekday nights customers came in earlier and left earlier. The Mineshaft was laid out on two windowless floors: the front entrance led to a blackwalled flight of stairs on which one waited on line, with one's eyes at the level of the small of the back of the person in front. At the top of the stairs stood a bouncer and an assistant manager behind a small lectern where one showed identification and paid admission. "Members" paid a lower rate than "nonmembers," but "nonmembers" were given a "temporary membership pass" which advised them of the Mineshaft's rules of admittance and decorum. These included a dress code which expressly forbade designer clothes of any kind, suits and ties and dress shoes, "drag," and cologne. It also applauded clothes associated in American culture with working-class masculinity: levis and leather, T-shirts, boots, lumber jackets and uniforms, and "just plain sweat." In practice, one would be refused admission for inappropriate dress, and in some cases the exclusion criteria were extended on the basis of unwritten rules by the employee at the door to judgments of appearance, deportment, or reputation as well. For example, attempts were made to exclude pickpockets. In general, it appeared that the exclusion criteria were applied fairly consistently to those wearing forbidden articles. If one was not a member, there was a greater chance of being refused admission. Memberships were sold at a variety of rates (for example $10.00 for three months) and entitled one to receive discount admission for the period in question. Membership meant one's name was put on a membership list, and a glossy black plastic membership card, the size of a credit card, was issued in that name. Members also recorded their "alias" or "code-name" while signing up for membership. These were typically masculine and informal such as "Butch," "Skipper," "Johnny Boy," or "Dick." This combination Boys' Club and pseudorationalized bureaucratic ritual may well have cosmeticized a genuine gatekeeping function defined by the need to circumvent legal authority.

The first room one entered after being admitted was the "front room." This was a large space, with spotlit pool tables, a long bar which was the most brightly lit area in the Mineshaft, a coat-check area, and a few benches in the shadows along the far wall. The walls were mostly unvarnished planks and there was sawdust on the floor, as there was throughout the upper floor. Near the front entrance was the entrance to a red-lit restroom which contained a number of stalls, urinals, and a small single sink which allowed water to splash onto the floor. At the coatcheck a sign offered a 5-cent discount to anyone who was "uncut and could prove it." Coatcheck employees were friendly and would without question check any and all articles of clothing a customer wished. This allowed some imagination to be used in devising appropriate costumes, since customers could check their street clothes and don something more exotic. One evening, for example, I was startled to realize that the man standing silently next to me in the shadows was wearing a New York City policeman's uniform. When I could speak, I whispered, "I think it's a raid," and was informed by someone nearby, "Huh? Oh. No, he always does that." On crowded evenings, a coatcheck line would form during peak entry hours, and again at closing. The coatcheck thus represented a second transition zone, one where minus the uncertainty of admission one could get into costume, or look around and stake out the territory. The front room was the most convivial area of the Mineshaft, as it was the only area where "talking out loud" was not frowned upon. It was a place to "get in the mood" for further activity, or to "relax" prior to returning to the outside world. People spending time in the front room were often willing to have friendly conversations, but the front room was also a favored place for initiating sexual contact. Scenarios that used verbal scripts to develop erotic momentum found a place here. Occasionally it became the scene for a variety of simple activities that used the pool table or the bar as props: people would bend over a pool table, sit astride or stand at the bar, while their partners would penetrate or fellate them. It was especially appropriate for those who enjoyed a sense of public spectacle, exhibition, or humiliation. Activities at the bar were somewhat constrained by the expectation that those standing there would order drinks. A sign over the bar listed the suggested "donations" of $1.00 for beer and $2.50 for liquor. If erotic activity began close by people whose conversation was unrelated to the activity, the talkers might move away slightly so as not to be in the way, they might ignore it, or, rarely, they might lower their voices and watch. The front room set a tone of noncompetitive respect for and indulgent nonchalance about sexual activity that became the rule throughout the Mineshaft.

Activities begun in the front room might also move into an adjacent area. The red-lit restrooms were often the site of watersports. A more dramatic transition was the darkened archway that led to the blackwalled "playground." The playground had its own set of rules which were spelled out on the temporary membership pass: no talking, no laughing, no dishing in the playground. Above the entrance another sign gave the more practical advice: No winter coats in the playground. The playground (and the entire lower floor when it was in use) were usually maintained at a higher temperature than the front room. It was much dimmer than the front room, contained a small bar, a table, some wooden stalls, two recesses which contained slings, and featured a spotlit wooden frame in the center with a sling about six feet off the ground. The slings were used to suspend men who wished to be fisted, and the bartender at the small bar would provide paper mayonnaise cups of Crisco and handfuls of paper towels to those doing the fisting. The wooden stalls could be used by those wishing to exclude others, but also had "glory-holes" to allow both voyeurism and pseudoanonymous fellatio. The table was moved about from time to time and used variously. One evening I observed a man lying on it while another stood over him dripping hot wax from a red candle on his nipples. The playground also had its own small restroom.

The lower level could only be reached through the playground, and was only open during the weekend crush. In effect, then, it was an extension of the playground belowstairs. Two flights of stairs went down. One, reached through a door, was a standard, wide, steel-reinforced stairway that presumably conformed to fire regulations. The other, spotlit and situated just behind the central fisting frame, was a ramshackle, single-width, barely navigable wooden staircase, which presumably looked appropriate to an abandoned mine. Customers did not appear to have any preference between the two stairways. The lower level was more extensive than the upper but was internally divided by concrete walls, which were painted black throughout. The first part of the lower level was virtually a maze. The floor was not level, and the area was difficult to navigate, pitchblack in some corners. Most of the darkened corners were the setting for ordinary fellatio or intercourse, between pairs or in groups. Beneath the wooden stairway were several more wooden stalls with glory-holes. In one section, kept especially warm, were several bathtubs. Men would sit in the bathtubs, usually naked, but occasionally clothed, waiting for others to urinate on them. The silence of this activity was occasionally broken by whispered encouragement. In another room was a stage, but I never observed it used for a performance. The last room on the lower floor contained a large bar, which was overshadowed by an enormous mirror in which one could observe the room as if from a bird's-eye view. This room was used primarily for "backroom" style sex, that is, whatever activity people wanted to engage in with those adjacent to them in the crowd.

The Mineshaft was equipped with a sophisticated sound system which was used to play original tapes. The tapes were eclectic, but favored avant-garde, punk, and classical music. The sound system operated at a lower volume in the front room than in the playground areas.

Role Systems and Ritual Drama

In spite of the complexity of the institutional, cultural, and psychological forces which appear to have been at play in the Mineshaft on a typical Saturday night, it nevertheless appeared that socially structured roles in the formal sense were rather simple. Since, at least from the customer's viewpoint, the meaning of a Mineshaft experience was a highly personal one, it was necessary for individuals to feel free to develop their own fantasies and create their own roles to match. Such personal improvisation was a form of self-education, and I would hypothesize, unlike Sambian initiation, was largely self-directed. I would suggest, however, that two simple role systems operated. These can be described as the distinction between employees and customers and between members and nonmembers.

The former corresponds to the capitalist political economy which created and sheltered the Mineshaft. From this perspective the Mineshaft was part of the American entertainment industry, and its employees provided a service. The distinction between employees and customers exists in any commercial organization. Like most employees in the ghetto, Mineshaft employees were workers in the secondary labor market, and dependent on tips.[7] They dressed like customers, fraternized freely with customers, and in some cases might become customers during their free time. This apparently vague line between the two roles was characteristic of ghetto employment, but was especially vague at the Mineshaft. This might have been partly a result of the relatively high complement of ghetto workers among the Mineshaft's clientele, whose expertise would make them demanding; and partly due to the Mineshaft's marginal legal status, which would make management wary of any overt conflict with customers. Since the municipal police were probably paid off to ignore the Mineshaft's existence, they could hardly be called in to deal with any altercation. Along with their manifest duties, employees would look out for the welfare of customers, who might, for example, require medical attention. They would eject pickpockets. On one occasion, I observed someone who had passed out being carried up the stairs.

The line between members and nonmembers was less formal than it sounds, and I have already suggested that it could be operationalized in a variety of ways, such as weekend versus weekday night attendance, or newcomers versus old hands. It has been described in a romantic short story about the Mineshaft (Preston 1984, p. 80) as, in effect, the difference between "The Committed" and the presumably not-so committed. The significant variation was one of degree of socialization.

Of course, the normative standards of membership in the Mineshaft did not assume any single definition of masculine erotic reality. Indeed, the ability of the Mineshaft experience to accommodate the individual homoerotic realities of hundreds, if not thousands of gay men, was its most interesting feature. While each participant performed his own ritual with his own meanings, the Mineshaft functioned somehow to hook up all these performances with a common set of facilities, rules, symbols, and emotions. It suggests on the one hand, the possibility of a nonviolent community in a fragmented, specialized, and culturally atomized society; or forces one to "consider the dionysian as an archetypal aspect inherent in every society" (Maffesoli 1983). Thus, in contrast to the two simple socially imposed role systems just described, ritual dramatic roles at the Mineshaft were flexible and complex. Nothing prevented an individual who so desired a variety of roles in any number of different activities, even during the course of a single evening. The lighting was dim, there was no reason to speak aloud, and one could change costume. Men who were tired of playing erotic subjects could find a way to be erotic objects, and vice versa. Some ritual activities, especially those involving more than two participants, were far more complex than simple dyads. Indeed, spontaneous orgiastic combinations centered on fellatio, masturbation, and anal intercourse were quite liminal. Even clearly defined active/passive dyads in the context of the Mineshaft were often transformed into group experiences, and informants have described their experiences in the Mineshaft as having had a religious meaning. For example, consider the following description of a playground whipping from Preston's romance:

> The men who crowded us couldn't help but try to touch him. Even while my belt thudded on his back their hands would reach out and worshipfully attempt to feel some part of him. They were awesomely silent. It was as though a new, precious icon had appeared in this house where men were venerated. (1984, pp. 82–83)

In this story the narrator decides that the man he is whipping does not really want these others around, that "it broke the finely tuned communication between us." So after an interaction wherein "he kissed me just a little," the restored dyad "go back to the front." "People followed us from room to room hoping that the ritual this man and I were performing would be repeated," reports the obviously boastful narrator.

As in this example, the main problem of social control in the Mineshaft centered on this tension among the tremendous variety of erotic fantasies people might be acting out in any given encounter. This tension was usually contained by an extraordinarily fine-tuned etiquette of glances, gestures, movements, and whispered encouragements or "dirty talk." During the entire period of observation I only witnessed one incident involving actual rage or violence, an exception which revealed the rule of ritualized social control. This took place on an especially crowded weekend evening on the lower floor in the superheated area near the bathtubs. A man called out very loudly "I said STOP THAT!" and apparently struck another man. The crowd was stunned, and in Goffman's terminology, the frame was obviously broken—no one knew what to do. All sound but the disco tapes ceased. People all around stopped what they were doing and stood frozen as if in a tableau. The man continued to shout and struck out several more times. It appeared to me that he struck out at random, and may have injured more than one person. Someone called out "Hey, no fighting!" One injured man left the area. Finally people close to the assailant began to take action appropriate to the situation, taking hold of the man and talking to him. The assailant was maneuvered away, while some of those who had witnessed the incident edged out of the area, clearly disturbed. Meanwhile newcomers moved in, and the frame was reestablished within a few minutes.

Conclusion

What then do we know about the Mineshaft?

Decoding the language of social control used in the Mineshaft would need systematic study of a similar site. Such a study would need to include such symbolic languages as costume, pose, and choreography. The boundary between the front room and the playground suggests Mead's discussion of the relation between games and play (1962, pp. 151–63). The Mineshaft fostered both intense play, where one took on a single role and played it, and the greater complexity of the game, where knowledge of other roles (and the roles of others) was also required. The Mineshaft needed to accommodate different levels of understanding of every language it used. If an initiate was unable to articulate his needs through costume, or moving in a certain way, or standing in a certain position, he might still be able to stumble upon fulfillment in the dark, or just stand still until someone with clever hands decoded his secret. The complex and ill-lit layout necessitated slow, stage-like movement, even when crowds were not present, and simultaneously facilitated fantasy.

But analysis must move beyond the symbolic; it must also examine touch, smell, taste, and nonverbal sound as nonsymbolic avenues of culturally meaningful experience. In a highly verbal culture, where words and mass-produced images dominate socially constructed reality, the dim lighting and primarily nonverbal communication of the playground eerily emphasized the openness of touch, smell, taste, and nonverbal sound as avenues of experience. These zones were as much a vacant niche in the psychocultural landscape of America as the meat-packing district in which the Mineshaft was located was a vacant niche in the political economy of the urban landscape. The playground especially was devoted to the way things literally *felt* to participants. It was a place where cultural inhibitions were displaced, rather than discussed; that is, an arena of critical practice, rather than critical discourse.

The Mineshaft may have addressed unarticulated and neglected desires of gay men for social sanctioning by allowing individuals to act out their fantasies and "unwind their reels" in a group setting. If so, how deeply did these experiences affect people? How did they interpret what was going on around them? How well did their experiences match the diversity of their fantasies?

The Mineshaft probably functioned to socially organize risk reduction at the nexus of the S&M and larger gay male communities by maintaining an environment in which limiting experimentation could be carried on in the presence of experienced persons. Relative to less organized alternatives such as the streets and dockside, it was a safe place for initiates into the S&M world to meet those with developed S&M identities. It was at times a site of awesome and liminal rituals of initiation which the culture in which it was situated maintained in secrecy and considered taboo. As was also true in the Sambian rituals, humiliation and fear were linked with affection and mutual erotic satisfaction.

At the same time the Mineshaft was not under the control of the homoerotic male community. It was clearly the creation of secondary labor market capitalism and maintained through traditional forms of political corruption. Its owners allowed its use as a vehicle for media exploitation of gay men.

Nevertheless, nightly, it clearly demonstrated the power of culture and social organization to transform sensation and physiological response into erotic experience.

Notes

1. Such as those between, on the one hand, normative ideals of "equality" and "freedom," and on the other hand, the realities of inequities of power and constraints on opportunity.

2. Liminality, and its relationship to *communitas*, is a central concern for Turner (1969). In a *rite de passage*, the individual or group undergoing the rite is first separated from social structure or cultural givens before becoming liminal, i.e., not subject to social definition, "neither here nor there" (op. cit., pp. 94–95). *Communitas* is the relatively unstructured society which emerges in the liminal phase. As will be shown, the Mineshaft could well have provided its customers with such experiences.

As a more classical example of ritual liminality it is interesting to note Herdt's (1982, 1987) discussions of Sambian initiation. The initiation experience, as Herdt describes it, is "deeply awesome" (1982, p. 68) if not terrifying, rather than "fun," although for the older participants it seems enjoyable enough. This difference between the experience of the initiates and that of the older males seems due primarily to the secrecy which is maintained about the rites, as a result of which the initiates have no clear expectation of what will happen to them.

During the ceremony, violence and joking hostility are exercised by the older males on the initiates, and a homoerotic norm is successfully introduced and established in most cases. This norm involves an explicit association between fellatio and flute playing, whereby the flutes are eroticized. The young boys are taught that performing fellatio on older males is necessary in order to become men themselves. They ultimately learn to enjoy this activity and enter into various libidinal liaisons with older men to whom they are attracted. The initiation also prepares them for their subsequent role as older participants in such relations.

A startling surface similarity between the Sambia and the United States lies in the secrecy attached to homoerotic socialization. However, the secrecy attached to the Sambian rites is hegemonic within the tribe, secret knowledge which is a source of power for its practitioners. In the United States the secrecy attached to homoeroticism is resistive, a result of domination.

3. The Mineshaft's decor, for example, was in some ways suggestive of a late evening at some of those outdoor sites in its vicinity at which many patrons would have erotic experiences under conditions of considerably greater personal danger of, among other things, being mugged. Certainly, as will be discussed below, the Mineshaft's location was as out-of-the-way and its admission policies as elaborate as anything necessitated by police surveillance during the early 1960s.

4. For example, the need to develop stigma management skills, or overcome internalized negative stereotypes of gay identity. This has improved somewhat in that there are now books available on how to come out to one's parents or maintain a long-term relationship with another man, and in large cities psychotherapists willing to help one develop a positive gay identity. But where does a fifteen-year-old go to find true love, or failing that, to practice sexual risk reduction techniques, with other young men?

5. A service economy centered in Greenwich Village had emerged

with extraordinary vitality from the underground during the previous decade. During the early 1960s as few as five packed gay bars might be serving the entire metropolitan New York area at a given moment, and these were subject to Mafia administration and police pay-off, and of course, raids. Even private gay parties were subject to raids. The "Stonewall Rebellion" of June 1969 was essentially a communal response to a bar raid, but marked the beginning of a new era of relative governmental indifference to nonpolitical group activities of gay men.

6. As Barry Adam has reminded me, there were also back rooms in some bars in operation during regular hours.

7. Secondary, relative to primary labor market employment, is characterized by low pay, low status, short or nonexistent career ladders, lack of benefits, nonunionization, job insecurity, and transience.

References

Adam, B. D. 1978. *The Survival of Domination.* New York: Elsevier.

Dynes, W. (1985). *Homolexis: A Historical and Cultural Lexicon of Homosexuality.* New York: Gai Saber.

Goffman, E. 1963. *Stigma: The Management of Spoiled Identity.* Englewood Cliffs, N.J.: Prentice-Hall Inc.

Herdt, G. H. 1982. "Fetish and Fantasy in Sambia Initiation," in *Rituals of Manhood: Male Initiation in Papua New Guinea,* ed. G. H. Herd, pp. 44-98. Berkeley: University of California.

———. 1987. *The Sambia: Ritual and Gender in New Guinea.* New York: Holt, Rinehart and Winston.

Kamel, G. W. L. 1983a. "The Leather Career: On Becoming a Sadomasochist," in *S&M: Studies in Sadomasochism,* ed. T. Weinberg and G. W. L. Kamel, pp. 73–79. Amherst, N.Y.: Prometheus Books.

———. 1983b. "Leathersex: Meaningful Aspects of Gay Sadomasochism," in *S&M: Studies in Sadomasochism,* ed. T. Weinberg and G. W. L. Kamel, pp. 162–74. Amherst, N.Y.: Prometheus Books.

Krafft-Ebing, R. 1965. *Psychopathia Sexualis,* trans. F. S. Klaf. New York: Bell.

Lee, J. A. 1983. "The Social Organization of Sexual Risk," in *S&M: Studies in Sadomasochism,* ed. T. Weinberg and G. W. L. Kamel, pp. 175–93. Amherst, N.Y.: Prometheus Books.

Maffesoli, M. 1983. *The orgiastic as an agent of socialization.* Handout at the conference *Among men, among women: Sociological and historical recognition of homosocial arrangements,* Universiteit van Amsterdam, June.

Mains, G. 1984. *Urban Aboriginals.* San Francisco: Gay Sunshine.

Mead, G. H. 1962. *Mind, Self, and Society,* ed. C. Morris. Chicago: University of Chicago. (Original work published 1934)

Murray, S. O. 1984. *Social Theory, Homosexual Realities.* New York: Gai Saber.

Newton, E. 1972. *Mother Camp: Female Impersonators in America.* Chicago: University of Chicago.

Preston, J. 1984. "Interludes," in J. Preston, *I Once Had a Master,* pp. 80–89. Boston: Alyson.

Rist, D. Y. 1985. "Policing the Libido." *The Village Voice,* November 26, pp. 17–18, 20–21.

Russo, V. 1981. *The Celluloid Closet: Homosexuality in the Movies.* New York: Harper & Row.

Spengler, A. 1983. "Manifest Sadomasochism of Males: Results of an Empirical Study," in *S&M: Studies in sadomasochism,* ed. T. Weinberg and G. W. L. Kamel, pp. 57–72. Amherst, N.Y.: Prometheus Books. (Reprinted from *Archives of Sexual Behavior* 6 [1977]: 441–56)

Townsend, L. 1993. *The Leatherman's Handbook II,* 4th printing. New York: Modernismo.

Turner, V. W. 1969. *The Ritual Process: Structure and Anti-structure.* New York: Aldine.

Weinberg, M. S., and C. J. Williams. 1974. *Male Homosexuals: Their Problems and Adaptations.* New York: Oxford University.

Weinberg, T. S. 1983. "Sadism and Masochism: Sociological Perspectives," in *S&M: Studies in Sadomasochism, ed.* T. Weinberg and G. W. L. Kamel, pp. 99–112. Amherst, N.Y.: Prometheus Books. (Reprinted from *The Bulletin of the American Academy of Psychiatry and the Law,* 6 [1978]: 284–95)

STRUCTURES
THE SOCIAL ORGANIZATION
OF S&M

Introduction

The article by Thomas S. Weinberg and Martha S. Magill examines how sadomasochism has now become integrated into the culture of mainstream society. The inclusion of sadomasochistic themes in recent mainstream magazine articles, comic strips, movies, television, fashion, art, and popular music is discussed as examples of how knowledge about sadomasochism is no longer confined to a hidden subculture, but is commonly known about and understood within American and similar cultures. Especially in the more cosmopolitan cities, sadomasochistic clubs are accessible to those who seek them. Sadomasochists appear on popular television talk shows and explain their ideas to a national audience. There are even seminars in dominance taught in adult education programs. And advertisers in meeting place ads in the daily newspaper often note their sadomasochistic interests.

While some ideas on identity and S&M scenes are included in G. W. Levi Kamel's discussion of "Leathersex," this contribution focuses primarily on sadomasochism as an organized subculture. Rather than view S&M stereotypically as randomly violent behavior, Kamel shows that it is a highly prescribed, normatively controlled, and rationally accomplished sociosexual activity. It is, in a word, socially *meaningful* behavior among its participants. Some of the tenets of existential sociology are implicit throughout the essay.

The contribution of Norman Breslow, Linda Evans, and Jill Langley is especially important, given the dearth of information on nonprostitute women in the S&M scene. Using a questionnaire placed in two sadomasochistically oriented magazines, along with responses gathered from those distributed by an S&M oriented shop and an S&M club, Breslow and his colleagues provide data on fifty-two women. They found that women recognized their S&M interests later than did the men in their study and that they were introduced to sadomasochism by others, rather than having recognized a "natural interest" from childhood. Breslow et al. also noted that these women were more active in S&M than were the men who also responded to the questionnaires.

Importantly, Breslow and his colleagues did not find any significant differences between men and women in their preferences for the dominant or submissive role, thus calling into question assumptions made by earlier writers such as Freud and Krafft-Ebing.

Rick Houlberg's work differs from the others in this collection, since it reports the results of a content analysis of the magazine of a sadomasochistic club. He views the magazine as a vehicle for creating shared meanings for club members. His analysis gives us insight into the history, politics, and social organization of the club through its official publication, while also providing information about the concerns of its members.

Thomas S. Weinberg and Martha S. Magill

Sadomasochistic Themes in Mainstream Culture

Over a decade ago, Falk and Weinberg (1983) noted that sado-masochistic themes could be found in many parts of popular Western culture, and that their appearance could be traced back to at least the mid-eighteenth century. Although Falk and Wein-berg presented examples of recent movies, music, and literature to support their point, in the early 1980s, S&M still appeared infrequently in mainstream Western cultural life. Times have changed, and S&M has come out of the closet and into the living rooms of Americans. No longer "the last taboo" (Green and Green 1974) nor part of a hidden "velvet underground" (Gagnon 1977), S&Mers have appeared on national talk shows to explain their lifestyles. However, this does not mean that most Ameri-cans have an understanding of S&M or that they accept it. Nor does it mean that they perceive various aspects of popular cul-ture as having anything to do with S&M. For example, in the mid-1980s, the senior author appeared with a sadomasochist on a regional talk show (Richard Bey's "People are Talking," broad-cast from Philadelphia, which was a forerunner of his current

Specially written for this volume.

nationally distributed shows). The audience, egged on by the host, was extremely hostile and unwilling to try to understand the S&Mer's point of view.

S&M and the Media: Magazines, Newspapers, and the Information Superhighway

In the 1990s, sadomasochism has been discussed seriously in national media, both in the United States and abroad. For example, *Cosmopolitan* magazine published an article on S&M in its November 1992 issue (Levitt 1992). Despite its sensationalistic title, "The Scary Lure of Sadomasochism," the essay was not designed to titillate. Although the writer, Shelley Levitt, quoted therapists and presented the psychodynamic point of view, she also cited sociologists and presented the viewpoints of S&Mers as well. While she referred to sadomasochism as a "perversion" and "bizarre," Levitt also acknowledged that S&Mers do not see themselves as sick, and that, "Most hard-core S-and-Mers are content with their sexual orientation" (Levitt 1992, p. 214). She also emphasized that much of S&M is fantasy and that it is fulfilling for those who play out these fantasies. Another article, which describes the author's experience in a Learning Annex class on dominance taught by an "internationally known dominatrix," appeared recently in *Vanity Fair* (Markoe 1993).

In England, the (Manchester) *Guardian Weekend* ran a detailed cover article, complete with case studies, on S&M (Kershaw 1992). The article was at least partly the result of the Spanner case, a nationally publicized court case in which sixteen men were convicted for consensual sadomasochistic activities. While no complaints were made to police by the "victims," "11 men received sentences of up to four-and-a-half years for assault; 26 others were cautioned for the offence, thought to be unique, of aiding and abetting assaults on themselves" (Kershaw 1992, p. 6). The Spanner case, Kershaw reports, "has become the most bitterly fought campaign in an increasingly trenchant battle between radical sexual minorities and libertarians in one camp and conservatives, including some feminists, in the other" (ibid., p. 7).

Kershaw cites Pat Califia's article, which appears in this volume, and presents the view of another S&Mer, Kellen Farshea, founder of Countdown on Spanner, who defines S&M as consensual sex play, which may include sexual fantasy. He also quotes an S&Mer who says that, "The fact is, S&M is controlled and responsible sexual activity. We have a golden rule that when the bottom (masochist) says enough, the activity stops" (Kershaw 1992, p. 7). These three examples indicate that S&M is being given a serious and fair treatment in mainstream publications. Another form in which S&M has appeared in the print media is in contact advertisements. Those interested in S&M no longer have to patronize adult bookstores to find specialty magazines oriented specifically to the S&M subculture in order to make contacts with other S&Mers. Mainstream publications, especially those in the large metropolitan centers such as New York City, Toronto, and San Francisco, contain ads that are explicitly sadomasochistic. For example, a recent issue of the *NYPress* contained the following ads in its Press Match personals:

26 Y. O. STRAIGHT CURIOUS GUY
seeks kind, dominant, attractive person to make me cross-dress and fulfill your fantasy. Call and tell me all about it.

BiWM, EARLY 50s
seeks M or F for discipline and fantasy fulfillment. Beginners OK.

AGGRESSIVE YOUNG SEXY BF
5'6" into RPG[1]/games/toys, seeks submissive only M/F. Spanking, crossdressing a+. Enjoy the scene. Let's explore all.

DOMINANT GERMAN GODDESS
Tall, striking, orders devoted affluent male to submit now! Permanent placement possible. Serious only need respond.

Many daily newspapers and local or intra-city papers now feature special sections in which people can place ads to meet others at a nominal cost. Not all of them are so explicit as the ads above, but a careful reading of some of them finds codes understood by those in the S&M subculture.

The December 31, 1993, issue of the British publication *Private Eye* presented a large ad for a movie, *Decadence*, which debuted in January 1994. The advertisement for the movie, which starred Joan Collins and Steven Berkoff, depicted a woman wielding a riding crop while sitting astride a man.

S&M themes even pop up in the comics. In a "BC" comic strip, a little ant asks his father, "Dad, can I go out and play with Spanky?" "Sure," his dad replies. "NO!" his mother shouts. "Why can't he go play with Spanky?" his dad asks. "Because Spanky is a little girl with a whip!" she responds.

A very recent innovation in making S&M and other erotic contacts involves the so-called "information superhighway." There has been a veritable explosion in erotic computer bulletin boards, through which subscribers to various services can make contact with others of like mind. The back pages of the nationally distributed *Computer Shopper* contain advertisements from several erotic clubs and services, catering to a diversity of erotic tastes. Movies and CDs with S&M themes can be purchased by mail, or downloaded by the computer eroticist.

S&M in Literature, Film, and Music

Explicit S&M themes in literature have a long history. John Cleland's *Fanny Hill, The Memoirs of a Woman of Pleasure*, was privately printed in 1749. The Marquis de Sade published *Justine* in 1791 and *Juliette* in 1797 (Weinberg 1994). Perhaps the best known work to the American reader of erotica is *The Pearl*, subtitled "A journal of facetiae and voluptuous reading." Attributed to Algernon Charles Swinburne, *The Pearl* consisted of eighteen issues, distributed among an affluent clientele between July 1879 and December 1880; the readership enjoyed reading serialized stories with flagellation themes, such as "Miss Coote's Confession" and "Lady Pokingham," as well as witty poems such as "Charlie Collingwood's Flogging."

In addition to these more "classic" works, two subgenres of erotica were especially common in the late nineteenth century. One type of work chronicles the adventures of a young nobleman or roué, who in the course of his gaining sexual experience often encounters an older woman or prostitute who introduces him to spanking, flagellation, etc. Another common work is a "girls' school" novel, wherein a young woman "suffers" endless exploits with clergymen, teachers, or adult authority figures. Both of these anonymously authored subgenres hearken back to de Sade's *Justine*. Generally written in a tongue-in-cheek manner, they present sexuality as playful (Magill 1982). Often, the same scenes appear in one "memoir" after another, merely changing the name of the so-called school or faith of the clergy. These scripts live on in the brutality of 1950s reform school movies, as well as in more recent films such as *Chained Heat*.

A recent book, which received a great deal of attention from the media, is *Sex*, by the popular culture icon, Madonna. Packaged in a sealed aluminum foil wrapper, and bound between aluminum covers, the volume featured Madonna engaged in sadomasochistic activity, in S&M costumes and in various states of undress.

Sadomasochistic scenes, and sometimes themes, have made the transition from books to film. Joseph Wambaugh's *The Choirboys* is one example, as is the Anne Rice (AKA Anne Rampling) novel *Exit to Eden*, released as a film comedy in October 1994, in which Dana Delaney plays a dominatrix. Most often, S&M is played for laughs, an indication that the screenwriters feel that clued-in audiences are knowledgeable enough about S&M to respond with appreciation. For instance, the recent film, *Naked Gun, 33⅓*, has a very brief sight gag in which a dominatrix "encourages" Det. Frank Dreben to continue contributing to a sperm bank. At other times, S&M is presented in films as cruel or menacing, as in *The Night Porter* or *Cruising*. This dichotomy is similar to that in which gays and their world are represented.

Some popular music and music videos contain explicit S&M

themes, as do the stage shows of rock performers. Videos by Madonna are cases in point. Depeche Mode's song "Master and Servant" and the Rolling Stone's "Under My Thumb" are other examples.

Sadomasochism in Art and Fashion

During the 1980s, media exposure, especially that in newspapers and magazines, gave wider exposure to S&M themes, creating a desire among the more "hip" or trendy urbanites to experience the "scene." Media reporting of celebrities "slumming" or visiting New York City's S&M clubs (see Brodsky's article on the Mineshaft in this volume), of slave auctions at S&M bars, and actual labeling of clothing and pastimes as S&M legitimized public curiosity. In the major cities, artists familiar with the various S&M subcultures began to document themes and lifestyles. Exhibition of the photographic works of Robert Mapplethorpe provoked intense debate in the U.S. Senate about funding alternative lifestyles.

Perhaps women have had the most exposure to S&M themes as both fashion photographers, such as Helmut Newton, and fashion designers, such as Gianni Versace and Jean Paul Gaultier, openly admit S&M as a creative inspiration. Although first seen in European fashion magazines, women in the United States were initially exposed to S&M in the 1970s fashion magazine *Viva*. Since that time, studded and leather fetish-style clothing has become common in such publications as *Vogue, Details,* and *Paper,* as well as in Britain's *The Face*. S&M themes were elaborated by British designers Vivienne Westwood and Malcolm McLaren. Jean Paul Gaultier, the creator of what he labeled "bondage pants," and Malcolm McLaren, the "Father of Punk Rock," created looks that are commonplace in any mall. Whether labeled "punk," "gothic," or 1980s "New Wave," the novelty and shock value have worn off as the clothing has blended into the mainstream. Recent S&M clothing styles include tight leather pants (from the late 1970s on, although Diana Rigg's "Mrs. Peel," who wore skin-tight leather outfits in the 1960s television series, "The Avengers," is always mentioned by S&M devotees), dog collars and studded wrist bands (from the early to mid-1980s), stiletto boots and heels (from the mid-1980s), Gestapo-like women's jackets (fall 1992), corselets (fall 1994), police-type caps, and thigh-high black stockings intended to be worn with miniskirts (fall 1994). A September 28, 1994, edition of CNN Headline News showed a human interest spot reporting on a party at New York City's Puck building sponsored by Mont Blanc pens. The party featured models in full S&M dress. Later, people on the street were shown pictures from the September issues of *Vogue* and *Allure*, which presented a revival of the work of Helmut Newton and others who used S&M motifs. Some of the respondents recognized the clothing in the photographs as S&M, while others had no idea of their meaning.

Since 1990, people have sought to further distinguish themselves by more permanent body adornment, such as piercings and tattoos. The latter is now gaining mainstream acceptance, although "piercing parties" are a thing of the recent past.

Conclusion

In the last several years, S&M has received greater attention within mainstream Western culture. This has been especially apparent in the leisure time and recreational parts of social life. As this occurs more frequently, it will probably generate less controversy. The other side of the absorption of S&M themes into popular culture, is that this cooptation will undoubtedly generate changes in the S&M world. Subcultures have a way of preserving their separation from outsiders and preserving their uniqueness by constantly changing their symbols when these get coopted and thus diluted. When leather clothing, studded belts, and wristbands, high spiked boots, and corsets can be purchased in mall boutiques and worn by people who are oblivious to their erotic meaning, they lose their specialness. As one S&Mer complained, "Now *everyone* wears leather!" Leather clothing no longer held the same meaning for this man because he could not tell who was into S&M any more. It will be interesting to see how the proliferation of S&M themes in mainstream culture affects changes in the world of S&M.

Note

1. "RPG" = role-playing games.

References

Falk, Gerhard, and Thomas S. Weinberg. 1983. "Sadomasochism and Popular Western Culture," in *S&M: Studies in Sadomasochism,* ed. Thomas Weinberg and G. W. Levi Kamel, pp. 137–44. Amherst, N.Y.: Prometheus Books.

Gagnon, John. 1977. *Human Sexualities.* Glenview, Ill.: Scott, Foresman and Company.

Green, Gerald, and Caroline Green. 1974. *S-M: The Last Taboo.* New York: Grove Press.

Kershaw, Alex. 1992. "Love Hurts." *The Guardian Weekend* (November): 6–12.

Levitt, Shelley. 1992. "The Scary Lure of Sado-masochism." *Cosmopolitan* (November): 212–15.

Magill, Martha S. (1982). *Ritual and Symbolism of Dominance and Submission: The Case of Heterosexual Sadomasochism.* Ph.D. diss., Department of Anthropology, State University of New York at Buffalo.

Markoe, Merrill. 1993. "Dominatrix 101." *Vanity Fair* (September).

Weinberg, Thomas S. (1994). "Sade, Marquis de (Donatien-Alfonse-François, Comte de Sade)," in *Human Sexuality: An Encyclopedia,* ed. Vern L. Bullough and Bonnie Bullough, pp. 526–27. New York: Garland.

G. W. Levi Kamel

Leathersex: Meaningful Aspects of Gay Sadomasochism

Data and Methods

Leathersex is visible for the social sciences by way of adult literature and homosexual meeting places. My own employ in an adult bookstore led to innumerable opportunities for exposure to S&M people. Leathersex publications were scrutinized regularly, and periodic analysis of related pornographic novels and photos helped to confirm findings. Sex ads pertaining to S&M were analyzed from prior research (Laner and Kamel 1977). When sufficient rapport could be established with regular bookstore customers, heterosexual and homosexual, taped interviews were conducted. Three years of conversational interaction in leather-oriented bars across the United States and Europe created an invaluable overall impression of leathersex. But the bulk of information for this research is the result of informal conversations while in the role of potential participant, an insider role genuinely expected of the newcomer by experienced leathermen.[1]

A revised version of an article which appears in *Deviant Behavior: An Interdisciplinary Journal* 1: 171–91, 1980. Reprinted by permission of the author.

Action: The Practices of the Leathermen

For leathermen, S&M refers to the desire for dominance and submission. Acting out impulses to dominate or submit is accomplished by any number of practices. Most activities revolve around four basics: restraint, humiliation, masculinity, and fear. These feelings as they apply to the leathermen are best considered from the gay sadomasochist's meanings of "masculine"/ "feminine" and "dominance"/"submission."

Leathermen see gay sex as all-male encounters, and S&M for them is the ultimate in man-to-man interaction. In our culture, we understand dominance as masculine and submission as feminine, without the need to qualify such terms. But among leathermen, submission is not equated with feminine; "male submission" and the feeling of "masculine submissiveness" are, for them, perceptions with no contradiction. With this in mind, it is likely that gay masochists have fewer identity difficulties than their straight counterparts. The heterosexual masochist represents a cultural contradiction—he is masculine, yet submissive to women. Unlike his gay counterpart, he usually finds the task of redefining masculinity impossible. The gay man, if only because of his homosexuality, has already redefined masculinity. He does not necessarily "lose his maleness," or "wish to be a woman." Rather, maleness is understood not always in terms of dominance; it can be submissive, too.

In an aura of masculinity, then, the S (master or sadist) will dominate, and the M (slave or masochist) is willfully dominated. Even though basically an illusion, a game, the S&M scene[2] is most satisfying for participants when these emotional desires are acted out. Again, the activities and desires most consistently mentioned during interviews and informal discussions; in literature, publications, and pornography; and in the content of the sex ads reveal the four basic themes of restraint via bondage; humiliation via language, physical degradation, and watersports; masculinity via leather and roughness; and fear via threat of violence and pain. Though by no means exhaustive, these themes are central to the interests and activities of the gay sadomasochist.

Restraint: Role Establishment

Bondage, or restraint, achieved through the use of ropes, leather devices of all sorts, chains, or even heavy equipment such as racks and stretchers, is often employed during a scene—often at the very beginning. A few U.S. and European cities have gay S&M bathhouse setups with every imaginable restraining device available, from simple finger cuffs to a sophisticated reproduction of the French guillotine. Bondage, as used in the S&M scene, serves to establish roles, to deprive the slave of his choice of activities, and to direct power to the master. As symbolized by restraint, the slave yields his freedom to another man.

Bondage may be found as a scene in itself and will take on different meanings when not used in an S&M relationship. Likewise, S&M is sufficiently independent of bondage that leathersex may proceed without physical restraints. In this case, according to Larry Townsend's *The Leatherman's Handbook* (1977, p. 66):

> S&M without bondage is the M's (the slave's) game . . . we deal with the possibility of his moving out of the encounter if it ceases to turn him on. For this reason, the S (master) is faced with an even more difficult task. He is deprived of full physical control, and must maintain his command by other than ropes, or chains, or straps.

Fantasy thus becomes the primary device restraining the slave, and he is made to feel that any attempt to leave the presence of his master would be in vain, and would only elicit more punishment. The M will usually test the validity of his restraint, and at the same time verify his imprisonment in order to maintain his fantasy. And in response to attempted escapes, the S will more firmly establish his dominance by way of activities that humiliate, "demasculate,"[3] or inculcate fear. With or without the ropes, physical or psychological restraints help to establish and maintain roles.

Humiliation: Role Performance

Humiliation is a key ingredient in most S&M scenes. Although humiliation may have certain meanings for sexual scenes outside of S&M, for leathermen it is the method by which they carry out their respective roles. In this sense, masochists are in the act of being slaves and sadists are being masters, when performing acts of humiliation.

The master uses many methods to humble his slave, but among the most commonly employed is verbal humiliation, which involves the use of degrading name-calling (e.g., "cocksucker," "punk," and "worthless slut"). In addition, verbal activity includes dispensing of harsh-sounding commands and using terms or phrases that threaten the slave's well-being. According to several experienced leathermen, not all degrading terms are erotic. It may take several encounters and discussions before the S will hit upon a "magic word" for his M.

> I finally figured out after two years with Frank that he loves to be called a "punk-sucker." I stand over him with Levis on, pinch his neck to let him know who's boss, and say, "Pull it out, punk-sucker." Now he comes before I do.

Verbal interaction, designed to demean the M and give the S a chance to use his authority, may be essential to an encounter. This can be illustrated in the following verbal construct:

S: Beg for it, slave.
M: Please let me have it.
S: Please what, you asshole.
M: Please, sir!
S: You'll get it, when I'm ready.
M: Please, sir, now.
S: Maybe I'll whip you first.

Derogatory names, commands, and threats of violence are all directed toward the M, in an attempt to satisfy his desire to be humiliated.

Another strain of degradation, less common than verbal abuse, is "kennel discipline," or demasculation and dehumanization of the M by treating him literally like a dog. Licking the master's boots, being led around on a leash, wearing a dog collar, and even being forced to eat from a dog bowl are all possibilities. In more involved relationships, the slave may even spend an occasional night at the foot of his master's bed. Kennel discipline can become so involved that it may, on rare occasions, carry over to nonsexual parts of a relationship. This is an example of what Weinberg, following Goffman, has referred to as "breaking frame," in a previous essay in this volume.

Watersports, the use of urination during sexual activity, is most often thought of as a sexual variance for its own sake, and indeed it commonly is (Ellis 1966, p. 87). But when applied to S&M, its purpose is to degrade the slave and "exalt" the master. The difference in meaning is that in the former use of watersports, there is erotic fascination with the sight of urination itself, with or without the desire to come into contact. But in the latter, the S&M scene, being urinated on becomes symbolic of being degraded, used, and worthless. Actually, many of the usual watersports activities that entail extensive setups and cleanup: scatology, enemas, and other "bathroom sex," pose a problem in S&M—that of breaking the established mood. For urination, mats, bathtubs, and enclosed back yards are most practical, since such settings are easily moved into and out of.

Masculinity: Role Definition

Leather articles are essential to some, of some importance to others, and of no importance to still others involved in leathersex.[4] Leather is, of course, a popular fetish in itself, but with S&M it can be a strong symbol of masculinity. More specifically, leather represents the outward manifestation of "butchness," roughness, and the macho image. It is most often black leather that is approved of in the social or sexual settings of the leathermen. For some men, it is the look of leather that makes it appealing, especially when worn by an attractive man. Others like the taste of leather. Still others are aroused by the feel of it—usually, but not always, when someone is in it. The degree of importance of black leather is extremely situational and may depend on what the leather object is, who one's partner is, and how that item is used. The most common articles of leather are cockrings (straps of leather that in some way constrain the genitals), jockstraps, belts, boots, whips, and straps (for restraint, to threaten violence, or to wear with metal rings), jackets, and mats, to name a few. Steel is less commonly used than leather articles and usually takes the form of studs, spike inlays in leather, or restraints, such as handcuffs or wrist and ankle clamps.[5]

Human sexual feelings are such that interpretation and speculation on the meanings of specific acts by individuals are open to a great many possibilities. To illustrate, consider an isolated event during an all-male sexual encounter. A masculine man clad in tight leather pants, stands macho-style over his slave; and, on command, the slave begins licking his master's crotch. A researcher stumbles upon the scene. Having been exposed to a diversity of lifestyles, he has a basic understanding of what he is observing; that is, he sees two men in an act of sexual expression. In lieu of running off in shock at the sight, he decides that his researcher's curiosity is piqued more than his heterosexuality is offended. He therefore remains hidden and, pulling out the pen and pad he carries, he notes an immediately observable phenomenon: Both men have erections. He interprets this, quite accurately, as an indication that both men are sexually aroused by this single act (i.e., one man licking the black, leather-clad genitals of another). At this point, our observer becomes aroused also, in an intellectual sense, and asks Why? From the standpoint of his own sexuality, the observer is not nearly so puzzled by the master's turgid state as he is by the slave's. The observer decides to explore possible explanations.

First, it may be that the slave is aroused only because he was commanded to do the act. His excitement is due to a commanding voice, not the act itself, not the leather, and perhaps not even his master. Further, he could have been commanded to do any number of things, and the result would have been the same, as long as he defined the command in an erotic way. Second, perhaps the arousal is due to the act of licking in the area of another man's genitals, with the hope of eventual contact. The leather is not only irrelevant, but a nuisance, and the command is only tolerable if he eventually gets what he wants most. A third possibility is that our slave is turned on because the leather he is licking is his master's leather. Without regard for what his S has on, he is still aroused by the clothes that represent his master's authority, dominance, and masculinity. Further, anyone in the same clothes who did not "own" him would not be as attractive. A fourth possibility is that for the slave the leather is a full-blown fetish, and in sexually defined situations such as this, it is the taste, smell, feel, or all three sensations that thrill him. He must prefer that someone be in the leather, but male or female, dominant or submissive, is not important. Yet another possibility is that the licking behavior itself makes him feel "like a dog," and no force, command, leather, or particular partner would affect his state of arousal. In this instance, it is his own activity that turns him on, most probably with the aid of fantasy.

Our researcher begins to realize that there is no end to the number of possible interpretations.[6] Only a candid question and answer period involving considerable rapport could reveal the meanings the slave finds in his own behavior. And even then, the interpretation would rely on the assumption that the slave is adequately in touch with his own feelings and desires.[7]

Fear: Role Maintenance

After an analytical look at sadomasochism among homosexuals, one is left with the impression that it is not born of a confusion of pain and pleasure, but rather of a redefinition of pain.[8] A sadist generally does not take pleasure in causing pain for the mere sake of the act. Nor is it pleasurable if his lover does not share the S&M definition of pain (Mass 1979). Likewise, the masochist who stubs his toe on an unruly sidewalk does not get an erotic charge. Painful accidents are painful, with no confusion whatsoever. The pain of S&M is defined differently because it is a method by which partners maintain their dominant and submissive roles. It is a means to an end.

The whip, for example, takes on a threatening meaning for the masochist, and when in the possession of the master, it signifies who is boss. Even if used only lightly, the feel of the whip verifies or maintains their respective roles. The administration of pain is not defined as doing harm to another, but as dominating another. How much pain is desirable or tolerable is a highly individual matter, but it seems to be far less than is commonly supposed.

The means by which pain is given varies, but one of the most common methods is spanking, or more precisely, "ass slapping." Arm locks, head holds, and the like are also common. Another example is that of the S who will place a lighted candle at the proper angle for his slave to receive its drippings, sometimes while blindfolded. Generally, as an activity becomes more extreme, it is practiced and mentioned less frequently until it dwindles into the realm of fantasy.[9]

One experienced M, in a discussion on pain, explained, "The skilled master is not one who knows how to give pain, so much as he is able to inculcate the fear and the threat of pain and violence." Extremes, of course, exist. By far, most gay men in leather are not interested in, and are indeed very cautious of, extreme behavior in their sexual encounters. More than other groups, they are aware of the potential dangers of S&M. Compulsive sadists and masochists, rare as they are, may have lessened the credibility of leathersex; and the ways in which such persons are exposed and excluded are among the next set of considerations.

Norms: The Mores of the Leathermen

The activities and emotions described above are those of a minority of persons, and the participants are as much aware of that fact as anyone. One result of this awareness is a group cohesiveness of sufficient strength to generate shared norms, which may be subdivided into contact norms, action norms, and relationship norms. These norms act to control membership, activities, and emotions in ways that are different from mainstream gay society. If it is the differentness of S&M norms that makes leathersex so misunderstood, then a discussion of these may clear up some misconceptions.

Contact Norms: Membership Control

While mainstream gays often shun leathermen out of fear, S&M men exclude certain groups themselves, out of a fear more justified. Although compulsive S&M types are rare and are not likely to be part of the bar scene, in the bathhouses, or responding to sex ads in underground newspapers, they nevertheless pose a real threat to leather society. One precaution is the avoidance of those who have no social recognition; thus, transients and strangers are avoided. Whereas most gays would be attracted to new faces in their midst, S&M men are more cautious. The street pickups, often found in larger cities, are less inviting for the leathermen than for most gay people; thus, hustlers are avoided. (An exception to the "no hustlers" norm may be among those masochists who answer massage ads in underground publications. But the "masseur" is presumed safer than the street hustler.) Finally, rumor of one extreme activity by an S and his reputation can quickly be ruined in a city, since those who violate known limits are avoided.[10]

A conversation with a new S&M contact may sound like a "stability test," rather than the usual small talk of most gay bar settings. The leatherman is generally more careful than his gay brothers about who he invites home. One interview with a young M revealed typical stability questions directed toward potential partners:

> My conversation with someone new sometimes sounds like a questionnaire. I find out social standing, how long he's lived

> here, what sort of work he does, if he knows any of my friends, how much he travels, and on and on. If he has nothing to lose by violating my limits, I leave him immediately.

Implicit here is the belief that the maintenance of good social standing is valued enough to ensure safety. Social standing is equated with stability. This serves as an excellent example of the belief in the strength of informal social controls in a setting where formal controls are nonexistent. By comparison, the brand of sadomasochism often found in straight society, such as forced sex, lacks self-imposed, informal social norms for its containment. It appears to have little membership or organization. Without benefit of mutual consent, regular meeting places, or notions of limits, straight S&M often surfaces for public view in cases of violent sexual acts, usually involving unwilling victims of physical force. The social control is formal—the police departments, courts, and hospitals. Further, the S&M actions of gay men are carried out in prescribed manners, whereas action norms are rare among heterosexuals.[11]

Action Norms: Activity Control

A visit to a large city leather bar would quickly reveal to an observer that the gay S&M scene is socially, as well as sexually, laden with symbolism. The leatherman's appearance will tell his story. More than other gays, the men in leather have a lot to say about their sexual leanings, and they are inclined to say it with what they wear (Fischer 1977).

Masters and slaves are most likely to wear Levis or leather pants, with the master more commonly in the latter. Based on their appearance, they might be compared to bikers and jocks in one bar; both of masculine image, but one more so than the other.[12] The slave often wears a hankie in his right pocket, the master's in the left. In parts of the East, the opposite is true. Although codes vary and are subject to fad, certain colors of hankies symbolize particular desires, and several hankies in one pocket can read like a porno book. One could, according to one standardized code list, expect to find some combination of the following preferences in a given leather bar: burgundy—bondage; yellow—watersports; light blue—oral preferences; dark blue—anal preferences; red—fist fucking; black—heavy S&M; orange—anything goes." These more precise symbols are likely to be found in larger cities and only in leather bars. Many gay people would be no more familiar than Mrs. Jones with such color symbols, except to understand the meaning of which pocket is used and the more popular blue hankies. Another understanding of the subculture is the dangling of keys from one's belt on the right or left; this means passive or dominant, respectively.

Black leather jackets and motorcycle boots are almost standard, but anything in brown leather is often considered poor taste. Some slaves wear leather collars, plain or studded. Other gadgets, like handcuffs, may be worn from black, leather-studded belts to signify desires. Such a description as this is far from exhaustive, and only those totally involved in the scene could keep pace with the constant local, national, or even international changes and modifications.

Perhaps the most important of the action norms is the setting of limits which is simply a determination of how far a person goes in a scene—what he likes and dislikes. The more experienced leathermen can accomplish this in initial bar contact conversations without destroying the mood of excitement and anticipation. The M introduces his limits in subtle or indirect ways, perhaps by briefly discussing past experiences he has enjoyed most. It is commonly the M who steers the sexual content of the conversation; in that way he prescribes the action. The wise S avoids statements that might commit him to activities that are beyond the limits of the M. If at some point the M refers to his new bar friend as "sir," it means more than submission; it issues approval and signifies acceptance. Then the S is free to respond in degrading terms to begin mood establishment, but typically not before. The intensity of erotic interaction increases when the S begins to tell the M what he will "force" him to do, but only after the slave has indicated the extent and extremes of his desires. Many gays have objected to this form of conversation on the grounds that such what-do-you-like-to-do interaction seems inappropriate to a meaningful sexual encounter. Possibly the real distaste for verbal exchange of this type is rooted in the fear that it makes gay sex essentially different from straight sex, since heterosexuals supposedly know who will do what to whom. But for those involved in leathersex, initial conversations of this sort add to—in fact, they often initiate—the erotic mood, and in effect the participants begin to have sex before leaving the bar. And again, initial discussion of preferences is necessary for the leathermen because the nature of their orientation yields a more diverse set of sexual possibilities. But while other gays avoid the what-do-you-like-to-do syndrome, the leathermen stay clear of direct or overt discussion of their tastes, lest they defeat the initial purpose of initiating eroticism.

Another key norm also used as a safety device during leathersex is the "time-out" period, which gives both men a rest, or is called when the action gets too rough. Both men have the right, by the use of subtle clues, to call time-out. For the M, time-out may be indicated by referring to his master's first name, or some other taboo behavior. The S might simply state that he will "grant" his slave a rest, when he himself wants a break. Any mutually acceptable verbal or physical sign suffices; but again, neither man wants to break the mood of dominance and submission, so low-key activities or verbal abuse may continue, replacing the heavier action. Most time-out signals take the form of behavior that *slightly* disrupts the established S&M mood.

Most masters claim for themselves the ability to distinguish a real "no" from one that means "yes" by the voice inflection. As one recalls, "A few times (my slave) has yelled 'no' loud enough for the neighbors to hear. . . . I usually get the message." And another S: "I can tell a real 'no' because the others sound fake. There's no 'no' like a real 'no'!"

One more specific S explains the difference this way: "The fake 'no' sounds more like a whine or a plea, combined with a facial look of agony. The real 'no' sounds serious, and the look is that of anger." I suspect, however, that masochists may accompany their real "no" with slight verbal mood disrupters, similar to those used to request time-out.

It is also interesting to note a norm of avoiding the authentic verbal abuses—those terms of a hostile heterosexual society such as "queer," "fag," or "swish." Dominance and submission for most leathermen is not so real that they lose sight of a more genuine mutual respect. Likewise, their sense of self-esteem remains intact, unharmed by their activities. Outside the sexual context, an M can still be hurt in a genuine way, and an insensitive S can still be hurtful of feelings.

The literature and interviews reveal that although role exchanges during an encounter are rare, because they disrupt the S&M mood, the most exciting S has also served as an M, and the best M is capable of the S role. It is common for an S to have once been an M almost exclusively, and most leathermen begin their sexual lives as slaves. The high degree of role exchanges (even with the tendency for M role preferences in general[13]) may make S&M partners more sensitive to each other's emotional, as well as sexual, needs. In fact, other norms, involving the way in which an S and an M relate to each other in non-S&M situations, are found to exist on another level. These are, for lack of a more precise term, the interpersonal mores of the leathermen.

Relationship Norms: Emotional Control

Perhaps the most surprising revelation about S&M sex is that many times it culminates in masculine gentleness, warmth, and affection. Interviews and most scene descriptions in literature support the norm of showing intimacy for one's partner after orgasm, which serves to give the encounter deeper meaning and gratification. One man used these words to describe his long-term relationship: "(He) has the rare ability to satisfy my need to be loved, and (my) desire to submit at the same instant. One without the other is incomplete. I have always equated the two feelings in fact, and never enjoy settling for less."

Unlike the "quickie" encounters for which some gay men are notorious, total S&M scenes take more time, by the complexity of the activities. They require more than the usual commitment and trust on the part of the participants. Much more sensitivity to the feelings of one's partner is needed, and leathersex demands by its very nature a more intimate knowledge of the other man. In light of these impressions, then, perhaps it is not so shocking that leathermen express "softer," non-S&M feelings during and after an encounter.

Related to the usual higher degree of intimacy is the interesting aspect of lover arrangements among leathermen. Discussions indicate that roles often break down completely in domestic affairs. There is little relationship between sex role and daily duties (Townsend 1977). S&M is viewed as a fulfilling game, one not always needed or desired, and usually not central to the relationship. The general gay objection to S&M sex as "only a scene" is not grounded in the fact that the term *scene* is redefined by S&M men as "desirable encounter"; it is only a game perhaps, but one that is meaningful for those involved.

Men of the leather scene may be better able to express physical attraction without confusing it with love. The leathermen will more likely recognize each other's presence when they meet in bars, even when sexual attraction has worn off. They seem well equipped to express the precise feelings they retain for each other and are less likely to keep each other guessing about the "meaning" of past sexual encounters. They appear free to exhibit emotion without conventional obligation.

Among serious lovers, the positive S&M relationship is seen as a "total relationship," a unit of complementary desires. The master and slave are two sides of the same coin and fuse to the extent that the term "role" is only a convenient label, meaningless in reality. The world of male homosexuals is often depicted as one of an endless procession of acts of sex, with little concern for person, location, or emotion. True or not, such a view does not seem applicable to S&M relationships. They appear to be among the most stable arrangements of the gay community, bound by considerable emotional and personal investment, and not simply by ropes.

Notes

1. While talking to leathermen in the adult book stores and in S&M bars of major U.S. and European cities, I expressed interest in the scene on a personal level and overheard usual public bar conversation. Within all-male cruise bars, terminating interaction is generally easier than it is in most other settings, so that I found no difficulty separating intellectual interest from personal intention.

2. There are two reasons why the word "scene" is applicable in reference to gay S&M activities. First, it is used by the participants themselves. Second, its use should suggest that these activities may be analyzed as a theatrical performance without loss of empirical grounding. This work is intended to be more closely tied to the development of existential sociology with an emphasis on the link between private meaning and the emergence of a scene.

3. An analysis of pornography suggests that demasculation among heterosexual sadomasochists means 'feminizing,' usually through forced cross-dressing. Among homosexuals it means being dominated by another man *as* a man and cross-dressing is rarely involved. Cross-dressing would destroy the entire meaning of the scene.

4. The term "leathersex" is used in place of S&M in serious books and publications (as opposed to pornography), but is not often used among gays themselves, except perhaps by the most experienced. While leather is strongly equated with S&M among both heterosexuals and homosexuals, it is not a necessary ingredient.

5. Most large cities, especially in Europe, have specialty shops for S&M items. Leather shops often are willing to fabricate sex items for S&M people.

6. I wish to imply with this scenario that sociological interpretations of social behavior that are based solely on empirical observation may be inadequate. Rather, interpretation, if that is our goal, requires extensive consideration of meanings.

7. Perhaps the most useful methodology for understanding the nature of our existence is the analysis of personal experiences as they occur in given situations. For a discussion of this, see Douglas and Johnson (1977).

8. For a discussion on the redefinition and management of pain, as well as an understanding of the importance of the experiences of the researcher as data, see Kotarba (1977).

9. This theme is reflected in the analysis of the four volumes of *Leather Bondage Techniques*, a series of magazines that mix erotica with serious information. No author is given.

10. The norm of limits is considered shortly.

11. It is more difficult to study S&M among heterosexuals because they remain hidden. As a result of the lack of social organization, norms have not emerged as readily. One important work on heterosexual S&M is Greene and Greene (1974).

12. I do not wish to imply that the mannerisms of the leathermen are more masculine than that of other gay men; only their appearance.

13. This tendency has been noted by Townsend (1977) and is reflected in the analysis of *Drummer* and *Package*, nonpornographic periodicals for leathermen. Further, most of the erotic literature is intentionally written to titillate slave fantasies. Leathermen themselves agree that participants prefer the passive role by approximately 3 to 1.

References

Ellis, Havelock. 1966. *Psychology of Sex*, 2d ed. New York: Harcourt Brace Jovanovich.

Douglas, Jack D., and John M. Johnson. 1977. *Existential Sociology*. New York: Cambridge University Press.

Fischer, Hal. 1977. *Gay Semiotics*. San Francisco: NFS Press.

Greene, Gerald, and Caroline Greene. 1974. *S-M: The Last Taboo*. New York: Grove Press.

Kando, Thomas M. 1978. *Sexual Behavior and Family Life in Transition*. New York: Elsevier.

Kotarba, Joseph A. 1977. "The Chronic Pain Experience," in *Existential Sociology*, ed. Jack D. Douglas and John M. Johnson, pp. 257–72. New York: Cambridge University Press.

Laner, Mary L., and G. W. Levi Kamel. 1977. "Media Mating I: Newspaper 'Personals' Ads of Homosexual Men." *Journal of Homosexuality* 3 (Winter): 2.

Mass, Lawrence. 1979. "Coming to Grips with Sado-Masochism." *The Advocate* (April 5): 18–22.

McCary, James L. 1973. *Human Sexuality,* 2d ed. New York: D. Van Nostrand.

Townsend, Larry. 1977. *The Leatherman's Handbook.* San Francisco: Le Salon.

Whitman, Frederick L. 1977. "Childhood Indicators of Male Homosexuality." *Archives of Sexual Behavior* 6(2): 89–96.

Norman Breslow, Linda Evans, and Jill Langley

On the Prevalence and Roles of Females in the Sadomasochistic Subculture: Report of an Empirical Study

Introduction

Sadomasochism has not been a popular area for empirical research. The bulk of information on the subject comes from the writings of early sexologists (Krafft-Ebing 1922; Hirshfield 1956; Ellis 1954; Kinsey et al. 1953) or from theoretical papers. Most of the theoretical writings have been produced by Freudians and neo-Freudians (Freud 1961; Sadger 1926; Deutsch 1930; Horney 1935; Bonaparte 1952; Menaker 1953; Panken 1967; Eisenbud 1967), although in recent years behavioristic approaches have appeared in the literature (Brown 1965; Marks et al. 1965). Since there are numerous theoretical perspectives and variations within each theory, it is impossible to make definitive statements about sadomasochism with any degree of certainty.

The literature primarily concerns itself with the etiology of sadomasochistic behavior. Not surprisingly, the Freudian and neo-Freudian perspectives concentrate on early infantile and

Reprinted from: *Archives of Sexual Behavior* 14 (1985): 303–17. Reprinted by permission of the publisher and the authors.

childhood experiences. Problems encountered in various stages of psychosexual or ego development are viewed as the roots of sadomasochistic behavior exhibited in adult life. The behavioristic approach is also predictable in its views on the etiology of sadomasochism. Various conditioned responses are considered the cause of an individual's interest in this form of sexual behavior.

Despite these different perspectives, most theorists agree on the absence of female participation in sadomasochistic activities. Krafft-Ebing (1922) believed that sadism was a perversion of normal male aggressiveness; since he believed that females were not normally aggressive, their interest in sadism would be rare, and when found was symptomatic of lesbianism. He considered masochism a more normal state for women, and this very normality raised the problem of detection. It was difficult to distinguish masochistic sexuality from normal female sexuality. Hirshfield (1956) and Ellis (1954) shared this perspective.

Freud (1961) wrote that women's natural state was one of "moral masochism." As women lived their lives in this state, there was no reason for them to become sexual masochists. Freud differed from Krafft-Ebing in the belief concerning the potential for women to become sexual sadists. Freud believed that women were as aggressive as men and, hence, could express this aggressiveness sexually. However, writers from the Freudian perspective have failed to investigate further the behavior of female sadists, concentrating on males instead.

The behaviorists have tended to incorporate investigations on the modification of sadomasochistic behavior with studies in fetishism. Females have not been included in these studies, primarily because they are not considered to be fetishists. Men learn to associate certain stimuli with sexual arousal because their genitals are external and thus states of sexual arousal or nonarousal are easily detected. Females have more difficulty recognizing whether they are sexually stimulated and so do not learn to incorporate extraneous material into their sexual fantasies (Gosselin and Wilson 1980).

Few empirical studies on the subject have been conducted,

and none have included women in the investigations. Litman and Swearingen (1972) placed an advertisement in an "underground" newspaper, which had a large personal section with sexually oriented ads, seeking masochists who engaged in extreme forms of bondage. They received thirty responses, three from women. Although they interviewed the three women who volunteered as having sexual sadomasochistic interests, the women were excluded from the findings.

Spengler (1977) conducted what is possibly the best empirical study on the subject. He sent questionnaires to men who advertised in sadomasochistic correspondence magazines in West Germany and distributed questionnaires through S and M clubs. He limited his study to men because "it is almost impossible to question sadomasochistically oriented women in the subculture; there are hardly any nonprostitute ads and very few women in the clubs. As a result, we investigated men only" (pp. 442–43). Spengler suggests that female sadomasochistic prostitutes should be studied because only through them do heterosexual males realize their sexual sadomasochistic interests:

> We consider the assumption that manifest sadomasochistic deviance among women is very rare (at least within the subculture) to be essential for an understanding of the situation of [male] heterosexual sadomasochists. Accordingly, sadomasochistic prostitution, which in part affords the sole possibility for realization of the deviance for this group, plays a special role. With regard to our unsystematic impressions, nearly all the subcultural groups among heterosexual sadomasochists exist in cooperation with prostitutes. (p. 455)

Gosselin and Wilson (1980) conducted a survey in England that was similar to Spengler's but that concentrated on seeking correlations between the behavior and interests of sadomasochists, transvestites, transsexuals, and fetishists. Although women were contacted for the survey, they were considered to be prostitutes, interested only in financial gain, and so the data generated from their questionnaires were not combined with those of the men.

While the lack of female participation in the sadomasochistic sex scene is one of the few areas of near agreement between early sexologists, Freudians and behaviorists, a number of texts, popular books, and magazines (Comfort 1972; Green and Green 1973; Hunt 1974; Byrne and Byrne 1977; Victor 1980; Wolfe 1981) include females in their descriptions of sadomasochistic sexuality. These publications seem oblivious to the preponderance of technical writings stating that there are no such women. The questions remain as to whether females exist in meaningful numbers within the subculture and, if so, how they resemble sadomasochistic males.

Method

The authors contacted sixteen nationally distributed, sexually oriented publications that catered either partially or exclusively to sadomasochists. It was proposed that the publications include a questionnaire in their issues. This was done to avoid a sample population composed solely of individuals who were motivated enough to place ads seeking contact with others. Only one publishing company agreed to aid in this research. The questionnaire was published in two of their publications in 1982: *Letters*, a monthly digest-type magazine, and *Sugar and Spikes*, an annual digest-type magazine. To increase the sample size, approximately three hundred advertisers whose ads appeared in *Latent Image* (1982), a sadomasochistic contact magazine, were sent questionnaires. *Latent Image* was chosen because of its relatively low number of ads placed by prostitutes and its high number of ads placed by single females and couples. Additionally, a small number of questionnaires were made available by shops and one club catering to sadomasochists.

Materials and Procedure

The questionnaire consisted of forty questions that sought to elicit information regarding demographic factors and actual participation in sadomasochistic sexual activity. The questions were phrased in the terminology of the subculture. For example, the terms *dominant* and *submissive* were used in place of the terms *sadist* and *masochist* (these latter terms rarely appear in sado-masochistic ads). Additionally, although the term *sadomasochism* (S and M) was occasionally used in the questionnaire, it was usually replaced by the euphemism *unusual sex*, which is fre-quently used in advertisements appearing in sadomasochistic contact magazines. Other jargon was also used, and when such terms appear in this report, they will be briefly defined.

In addition to the forty questions, the respondents were asked to participate in a follow-up questionnaire, which con-tained twenty-one in-depth structured questions and a number of unstructured questions based on the answers to the original questionnaire. Approximately 50% requested to be included in the follow-up group, but only about half of these actually returned the second questionnaire. The responses to the in-depth questionnaire ranged from short, somewhat abbreviated answers to ten thousand to fifteen thousand word essays.

Results

Sample Population

There were 182 individuals who responded to the questionnaire. The majority of the respondents were from the United States; only twelve were not (6 were from Canada, 2 each from England and Italy, and 1 each from Sweden and Germany). Males num-bered 130 (72%), and females numbered 52 (28%). In response to the question, "Are you a professional dominant or submissive [sadomasochistic prostitute]?" 12 females (23% of females) and 10 males (7.7% of males) responded affirmatively.

Although the bulk of the literature would predict otherwise, a 1 x 2 chi square comparing the number of nonprostitute females to female prostitutes showed that nonprostitute females were represented in significantly larger numbers than female prostitutes (df = 1, χ^2 = 15.07, p < .001). Because of the relatively small sample of prostitutes, only the responses from the non-prostitute males and females are reported below. Table 1 contains general demographic data. No significant differences were found for the age distribution between the two groups of respondents. Significant results were found for levels of education, with males having reached a higher level of education than females (df = 4, χ^2 = 11.25, p < 0.05). A comparison with the 1981 Bureau of the Census figures shows that both groups are better educated than the population as a whole. These findings that individuals involved in the sadomasochistic subculture generally have reached a higher level of education than would be expected from the census figures are in keeping with the data reported by Spengler (1977).

Table 2 shows the marital status of the respondents. No significant differences in marital status were found between the two groups of respondents. However, when compared with the 1981 Bureau of the Census figures, this sample population was found to have different rates of marriage and divorce: they tended to marry less often or remain single longer, and those who did marry had higher divorce rates than the general population (males: df = 2, χ^2 = 20.88, p < 0.001; females: df = 2, χ^2 = 10.08, p < 0.0). One interpretation of this finding (Hunt 1974) is that individuals engaged in sadomasochism are personality disordered and unable to engage in meaningful relationships. An alternate hypothesis is that individuals engaged in sadomasochistic lifestyles do not do well in relationships where the other partner does not share his or her sexual interests. A number of respondents reported that this was the case. Other divorced but remarried respondents reported that their current spouses introduced them to sadomasochism and that they now find both their sexual relationship and marriage more enjoyable.

Table 1. General Demographic Data

	Male (%)	Female (%)
Age[a]		
25 and under	15.4	19.5
26–30	14.6	26.8
31–40	42.7	39
41–50	20.5	17
51 and over	6.8	0
N	117	40
X	36.2	33.4
S	9.96	7.73
Education		
Some high school or less	5.9	8.9
High school graduate	10.2	26.7
Some college	30.5	35.5
College graduate	31.4	20
Post-graduate	22	8.8
N	118	45
X	3.5	2.93
S	1.12	1.09
Monthly income		
$1000 or less	24	50
$1001–2000	38.5	13.3
$2001–3000	25.1	26.7
$3001–4000	8.6	6.7
$4001 or over	3.8	3.3
N	104	30
X	2031	1560
S	1426	1142

[a]These frequencies are the same as those used by Spengler (1977).

Table 2. Marital Status of Sample

Status	Male (%)	Female (%)
Never married	34.1	20
Married[a]	52.5	57.5
Divorced or separated	13.3	22.5
N	120	40

[a]Combined scores of individuals answering affirmatively as being either married or divorced but remarried.

Table 3. Significant Others' Knowledge

Knowledge	Male (%)	Female (%)
No[a]	25	2.6
Yes	75	97.4
N	104	38

[a]Combined data of those responding "No" and "I don't know"

Visibility

Respondents were asked whether their spouses or current boy or girl friends were aware of their sexual interests. Of the four choices—"No," "Yes," "I'm not sure," and "I do not have a spouse or current boy or girl friend"—the two categories *no* and *I'm not sure* were combined, since each indicated that the respondent was being less than open about his or her sexual interests (Table 3). The category indicating no present significant other was not included in this statistical analysis. These data reveal that the subjects are very open about their sexual interests with their significant others. Separate squares for each group of respondents revealed that both groups were significantly open (males: df = 1, χ^2 = 26, p < 0.001: females: df = 1, χ^2 = 34.1, p < 0.001). A comparison between the results of this question and that of Spengler (1977) cannot be made because he uses the two

Table 4. Age of First Interest

Age	Male (%)	Female (%)
6 years or younger	9.2	2.7
7–10	12.8	2.7
11–14	31.2	16.2
15–18	24.8	21.6
19–22	9.2	16.2
23–26	6.4	8.1
27–30	3.7	18.9
over 30	2.8	13.5
N	109	37
X	14.99	21.58
S	6.79	8.17

categories *knows or suspects* and *does not know*. *Knows or suspects* does not differentiate between those who are open about their interests and those who are not.

Age of First Interest

The respondents were asked to give the age when they first realized that they had sadomasochistic interests (Table 4). Males recognized their interests significantly earlier than females, as revealed by a 2 x 8 chi square (df = 7, χ^2 = 22.40, p < 0.01). Of the males, 53.2% realized they had sadomasochistic interests by the age of fourteen, compared to only 21.6% of females who realized their interests by that age.

Means of First Exposure to Sadomasochism

Respondents were asked to indicate how they became interested in sadomasochism (Table 5). A belief exists within the subculture that sadomasochistic interests are "natural ones" from childhood, that is, that they are the earliest sexual thoughts that can be remembered.

Table 5. Means of First Exposure

First exposure	Male (%)	Female (%)
Through reading pornography	21.3	17.6
From legitimate movies, TV, etc.	3.7	0
Introduced by another person	8.36	61.8
Natural interest from childhood	63.9	20.6
Other[a]	2.8	0
N	108	34

[a]This category has been deleted from the statistical analysis.

The data from Table 5 and those from Table 4 show that this may be true for some individuals but certainly not for all. Males did tend to feel that their interests were "natural from childhood" (df = 3, χ^2 = 139.2, p < 0.001). For computational purposes, the category *other* in Table 5 was deleted from the analysis. Although the males did feel that their interests were natural ones, the issue becomes clouded by the manner in which different men defined *childhood*. Older men (those in their fifties and beyond) tended to extend childhood to include their mid-twenties, while younger men tended to restrict childhood to the teenage years or younger. The females were seemingly introduced to sadomasochism by another person, although no significant results were found. Pornography, although a factor, is not a significant issue.

Participation in Sadomasochistic Subculture

Sadomasochists have difficulties meeting others who share their interests. Meeting places tend to be either nonexistent or difficult to locate. Moreover, sadomasochists do not necessarily appear, by dress or other means, different from the general population. How, then, do sadomasochists make contact with others who share their interests?

The respondents were asked to indicate all the means they

Table 6. Methods of Making Contact

Method	Male (%)	Female (%)
Through ads	40.6	41.7
At S and M bars	5.3	4.2
At S and M clubs	5.3	6.2
Seducing others	26.5	20.8
Have not tried	16.5	16.7
Other[a]	5.9	10.4
N[b]	170	48

[a]This category has been deleted from the statistical analysis.
[b]Indicates number of responses not number of responders.

used to meet others interested in sadomasochism (Table 6). Placing or answering ads in sadomasochistic contact magazines rated the highest for both groups of respondents. The second most frequent method was to introduce a sexual partner to sadomasochistic sex. Although about 17% of both respondent groups stated that they had not tried to meet others, this statistic is somewhat misleading. A number of respondents stated that they were introduced to sadomasochism by their present sexual partner and have no need to find other contacts. Others (usually females) stated that their current sexual partner found additional sexual partners (for group sex) and so replied that *they* had not tried to find others.

Number of Partners

Table 7 shows the frequency distributions of the number of different sadomasochistic partners during the year preceding the survey. The highest number of different partners was reported by females (mean = 8.6); heterosexual males reported the fewest number of different partners (mean = 2.9). This may be explained by an imbalance of the number of females to males in the subculture.

Table 7. Number of Different Sadomasochistic Contacts
during the Previous 12 Months

Partners	Male (%)	Female (%)
None	15.4	7.1
1–5	73	57.1
6–10	6.8	7.1
11–15	1.7	14.2
16–20	.85	3.6
More than 20	2.6	10.7
N	117	28
X	3.47	8.6
S	6.63	13.8

Table 8. Number of Different Sadomasochistic Sexual Encounters
during the Previous 12 Months

Encounters	Male (%)	Female (%)
None	12	9.7
1–10	43.5	25.8
11–20	16.6	19.4
21–30	11.1	3.2
31–40	0	3.2
41–50	4.6	12.9
More than 50	12	22.6
N	108	31
X	25	53
S	44.1	79.92

*Frequency of Sadomasochistic Sexual Activity
during the Previous Year*

Because of low expected values, no chi-square test between the
two groups is possible. From the means, however, we see that
females engage in sadomasochistic activity at a rate about twice
that of males (Table 8). The relatively low number of individuals
who have not engaged in sadomasochistic sexual activity indi-

Table 9. Sex Role Preference

Preference	Male (%)	Female (%)
Dominant	21	15
Usually dominant	12	12.5
Versatile	26	32.5
Usually submissive	14	18
Submissive	27	22
N	117	40
X	2.07	2.12
S	.86	.82

cates that those interested in finding others are capable of doing so. While Spengler (1977) found that 85% of his heterosexual male sample did not have sadomasochistic relations during the preceding twelve months of his survey, only 13.3% of the male heterosexual respondents in this study reported no encounters.

Sadomasochistic Role Preference

The respondents were asked to indicate their preferences for sadomasochistic roles (Table 9). For computational purposes, the categories *dominant* and *usually dominant* were combined, since usually dominant implies a preference for dominance. Similarly, the categories *usually submissive* and *submissive* were combined. *Versatile* denotes an individual who enjoys equally the dominant and submissive roles. A 2 x 3 chi square comparing males and females revealed no significant differences in role preferences between the sexes; nor did 1 x 3 chi squares reveal any preferences within each group. These data indicate that both male and female sadomasochists are equally distributed among the possible roles within the subculture. A small majority of both groups (males, 52%; females, 63%) either habitually or occasionally switch roles, while a large minority (males, 48%; females, 37%) state that they are inflexible.

The respondents were asked to indicate their sex role prefer-

Table 10. Sexual Orientation

Orientation	Male (%)	Female (%)
Heterosexual	61.1	42.1
Usually heterosexual	18.6	15.8
Bisexual	13.6	31.6
"Forced" bisexual	5.1	7.9
Usually homosexual	1.7	0
Homosexual	0	2.6
N	118	38
X	1.22	1.45
S	.46	.55

ence (Table 10). For computational purposes, the categories of *heterosexual* and *usually heterosexual* were combined, since usually heterosexual implies a preference. Similarly, the categories *usually homosexual* and *homosexual* were combined, as were the categories *bisexual* and *forced bisexual*. (A forced bisexual is an individual who enjoys homosexual sex only when bound or "ordered" to participate by a dominant/sadist.)

Both males and females in this sample showed a preference toward heterosexuality (males: df = 2, χ^2 = 70, $p < 0.001$; females df = 2, χ^2 =21.5, $p < 0.001$). Males tended to be predominantly heterosexual, while females tended to lean toward bisexuality.

Level of Commitment to Sadomasochistic Subculture

The respondents were asked to report the importance of sadomasochism in their lives: foreplay, lifestyle, fluctuating, or other (Table 11). For computational purposes, the category other was deleted from this analysis. Significant results were revealed for both groups, who viewed sadomasochism as vacillating between foreplay and a lifestyle (males: df = 2, χ^2 = 40, $p < 0.001$; females: df = 2, χ^2 = 9.88, $p < 0.01$).

Table 11. Level of Commitment to Sadomasochistic Lifestyle

Commitment	Male (%)	Female (%)
Foreplay	26.5	41
Fluctuating	58.1	43.6
Lifestyle	7.7	12.8
Other[a]	7.7	2.6
N	108	38
X	1.79	1.71
S	.58	.69

[a]This category has been deleted from the statistical analysis.

Table 12. Self-acceptance

Self-acceptance	Male (%)	Female (%)
Always	1.7	0
Often	2.6	15.4
Sometimes	23.1	15.4
Rarely	30.7	28.2
Never	41.9	48.7
N	117	39
X	2.68	2.69
S	.55	.61

Self-Acceptance

The respondents were asked to estimate how frequently they felt "dirty" or "perverted" because of their sexual interests: 1 x 3 chi squares for both groups revealed a high level of self-acceptance on the part of the respondents (Table 12). The most frequent response from both groups was *never*, which indicates a high level of acceptance of sexual orientation (males: df = 2, χ^2 = 108.5, $p < 0.001$; females, df = 2, χ^2 = 44.5, $p < 0.001$). This attitude of self-acceptance was also found by Spengler (1977) in his sample of males. For computational purposes, the categories *always* and *often* were combined, as were the categories *rarely* and *never* in this analysis.

Preferences of Sadomasochistic Sexual Practices

Table 13 shows the preferences of sexual activities of the respondents. The more extreme forms of sexual activity usually associated with sadomasochism, such as torture and activities involving excrement, are relatively rare. It is of interest that many of the sexual practices are enjoyed to approximately the same degree by both men and women (e.g., humiliation: males 65%, females 61%; spanking: males 79%, females 80%; masturbation: males 70%, females 73%; master-slave relationships: males 79%, females 76%). Females gave higher ratings to bondage, stringent (extreme) bondage, and restraint (mild bondage) than did males. Moreover, such "fetishes" as erotic lingerie and boots and shoes, always associated with males (regardless of the presence of a sadomasochistic orientation), were also rated higher by females as a sexual interest. Only the "fetishistic" interests in rubber/leather were shared equally by both sexes. Although much attention in the fantasies submitted by respondents was given to the feminization of males, only a few respondents indicated an interest in either transvestism or "petticoat punishment" (a form of transvestism in which the male is made to look ridiculous instead of feminine).

Discussion

The preponderance of the literature denies the existence of nonprostitute females in the sadomasochistic subculture. Accordingly, the subculture is viewed as predominantly homosexual, with the few heterosexual males relegated to the use of female prostitutes to realize their sexual interests. The data generated by this research contradicts this previous characterization of the sadomasochistic subculture. Nonprostitute females do participate in sadomasochistic sex, and heterosexual males are capable of making contact with them. This research revealed several similarities and differences between nonprostitute males and nonprostitute females.

Table 13. Preferences of Sadomasochistic Sexual Interests
(Sexual Interests of Females Compared to Males, in Descending Order)

Interest	Male (%)	Female (%)
Spanking	79	80
Master-slave relationships	79	76
Oral sex	77	90
Masturbation	70	73
Bondage	67	88
Humiliation	65	61
Erotic lingerie	63	88
Restraint	60	83
Anal sex	58	51
Pain	51	34
Whipping	47	39
Rubber/leather	42	42
Boots/shoes	40	49
Verbal abuse	40	51
Stringent bondage	39	54
Enemas	33	22
Torture	32	32
Golden showers	30	37
Transvestism	28	20
Petticoat punishment	25	20
Toilet activities	19	12

Similarities of Nonprostitute Males and Females

Both groups have large heterosexual and bisexual components. They fall within similar age ranges; males and females tended to be better educated and either to remain unmarried or to have a higher divorce rate than the population as a whole. While females made less money than males, the differences are similar to those of the population as a whole. Both are open about their sexual interests with their significant others; placing or answering ads and introducing sexual partners to sadomasochistic sex are the means by which both groups most often try to find partners. Both groups tended to be slightly submissive, although not significantly so. Both view sadomasochism as sexual foreplay, with interim periods of more intense involvement; both appear to think positively of themselves in relation to their interests in sadomasochism. Both males and females show approximately the same degree of interest in a large number of specific sexual acts.

Differences in Nonprostitute Males and Females

Males realized their sexual interests in sadomasochism considerably earlier in life than females. Males seemed to discover sadomasochism on their own, whereas females tended to be introduced to it by a sexual partner. Females engaged in sadomasochistic sex more often and tended to have a slightly larger number of different partners than males.

Conclusions

Having found that nonprostitute females do exist in the sadomasochistic subculture, although possibly in fewer numbers than nonprostitute males, further research in this area is indicated. Additionally, although the number of prostitutes in this sample was too small for meaningful analysis, an investigation into the similarities and differences between prostitute and nonprostitute sadomasochists is felt to be essential to an understanding of the subculture.

References

Bonaparte, M. 1952. "Some Biophysical Aspects of Sadomasochism." *International Journal of Psychoanalysis* 33 (4): 373–83.

Brown, J. 1965. "A Behavioral Analysis of Masochism." *Journal of Experimental Research Perspectives* 1: 65–70.

Byrne, D., and L. Byrne. 1977. *Exploring Human Sexuality.* New York: Harper & Row.

Coburn, J. 1977. "S&M." *New Times* 4 (February): 43–50.

Comfort, A. 1972. *The Joy of Sex.* New York: Crown..

Deutsch, H. 1930. "The Significance of Masochism in the Mental Life of Women." *International Journal of Psychoanalysis* 11: 48–60.

Eisenbud, R. J. 1967. "Masochism Revisited." *Psychoanalysis Review* 54: 5–26.

Ellis, H. 1954. *Psychology of Sex.* New York: Garden City Books.

Freud, S. 1961. *The Economic Problem of Masochism,* vol. 19, 1924; *Beyond the Pleasure Principle,* vol. 18, 1920, *Standard Edition Complete Psychological Works.* London: The Hogarth Press.

Gosselin, C., and G. Wilson. 1980. *Sexual Variations.* New York: Simon & Schuster.

Green, G., and C. Green. 1973. *S&M: The Last Taboo.* New York: Grove Press.

Hirshfield, M. 1956. *Sexual Anomalies.* New York: Emerson Books

Horney, K. 1935. "The Problem of Feminine Masochism." *Psychoanalysis Review* 22: 241–57.

Hunt, M. 1974. *Sexual Behavior in the 1970s.* Chicago: Playboy Press.

Kinsey, A., W. Pomeroy, C. Martin, and P. Gebhard. 1953. *Sexual Behavior in the Human Female.* Philadelphia: W. B. Saunders.

Krafft-Ebing, R. 1922. *Psychopathia Sexualis,* ed. F. J. Rebman. New York: Physicians and Surgeons Book Co.

Litman, R., and C. Swearingen. 1972. "Bondage and Suicide." *Archives of General Psychiatry* 27: 80–85.

Marks, I., S. Rachman, and M. Gelder. 1965. "Methods for Assessment of Aversion Treatment in Fetishism with Masochism." *Behavioral Research Therapy* 3: 256–58.

Menaker, E. 1953. "Masochism—A Defense Reaction of the Ego." *Psychoanalysis Quarterly* 22: 205–20.

Panken, S. 1967. "On Masochism, A Reevaluation." *Psychoanalysis Review* 54: 135–49.

Sadger, J. 1926. "A Contribution to the Understanding of Sadomasochism." *International Journal of Psychoanalysis* 10: 484–91.

Spengler, A. 1977. "Manifest Sadomasochism of Males: Results of an Empirical Study." *Archives of Sexual Behavior* 6: 441–55.

Victor, J. 1980. *Human Sexuality: A Social Psychological Approach.* Englewood Cliffs, N.J.: Prentice-Hall.

Wolfe, L. 1981. *The Cosmo Report.* New York: Arbor House.

Rick Houlberg

The Magazine of a Sadomasochism Club: The Tie That Binds

The study of sadomasochism has only recently emerged as a legitimate endeavor for social researchers. Weinberg (1987) stated: "It was not until the late 1970s that a body of sociological research on S&M began to appear" (p. 51). Weinberg goes on to note that earlier published research focused on sadism and masochism as individual pathologies and not as interactions between people. Recent publications, Weinberg argues, differ in issues addressed and in methods used but have as a unifying theme that S/M is "dependent upon meanings, which are culturally produced, learned, and reinforced by participation in the S&M subculture" (pp. 51–52). It is the social subcultures of S/M that are now receiving some study (Breslow, Evans, and Langley 1985, 1986; and Naerseen, Hoogveen, and Zessen 1987).

The S/M social subculture of this study is a West Coast sadomasochism club. The Club has over seven hundred members in two West Coast chapters, and almost one hundred other members scattered across the United States, Europe, and Australia.

© 1993, Haworth Press, Binghamton, New York. *Journal of Homosexuality* 21 (1/2): 167–83.

The Club produces a monthly magazine, and in each issue the Club's manifest is detailed. In addition to educating the public in the "understanding, interpretation, and appreciation of erotic art by providing commentary and literary review of eroticism in the arts," the Club will conduct lectures and group discussions in order to foster "the development of understanding and appreciation of erotic art" and the improvement of communication between erotic artists and the public. Finally, the Club provides instruction in the use of interpersonal erotic "psychodrama as a means to explore, share, and express erotic fantasy." The Club's statement of purpose also indicates the organization is self-proclaimed as the "second-oldest group of its type in the United States." In discussions with the author, the Club's founders indicated they thought only one New York City organization had preceded the Club.

The only "cardinal" rules which the Club's membership insists each member must uphold are that all S/M activities must be consensual, nonexploitative, and safe. As children are not considered to be able to consent, all activities must be between adults. The consensual and safety rules of the Club are constantly being reinforced. Safety and etiquette issues, including restrictions on overt and heavy drug use, are strongly stressed at new-member orientations and in all written materials produced by the Club.

Perhaps the most concise and articulate expression of the Club function was written by one of the Magazine's editors in 1986:

> Importantly, sexual and/or practice preference was not and is not a criterion for admission to [Club] membership. We have always had a gay, lesbian, hetero, bi, TS [transsexual], TV [transvestite], B&D [bondage and discipline], D&S [dominance and submission], infantilist, scatologist, etc., mix in [the Club]. One needed only a personal, nonjudgmental, supportive interest in safe, consensual, nonexploitative S&M activities.

The Club's Magazine

This study focuses on the Club's Magazine as a means of understanding the subculture represented within the Club. The Magazine is a periodic, primarily monthly, print publication which contains letters, stories, reports, poems, and photographs from Club members; financial, membership, and business meeting actions; reports from Club officers; and material from non-members such as reprints of newspaper articles and reports from other S/M organizations.

The publication was selected for study because: (a) the Magazine is the only recorded organizational history containing records such as membership reports and business meeting actions; (b) the publication provides a mediated forum for reflecting the S/M interests of Club members (stories, poems, photographs, interviews, etc.); (c) major conflicts within the Club, such as resource allocation and the dominance of one chapter over another, are played out in the Magazine; (d) approximately 15% of the Club's members reside more than one hour's drive from the two West Coast chapters and the publication is their only contact with the Club; and (e) the Magazine's editor is an important gatekeeper and an officer of the Club. Two other types of print media are also created by the Club: Printed flyers for special events such as parades and parties are occasionally mailed to Club members. A calendar of upcoming events was contained in an approximately monthly publication which was separate from the Magazine. At the end of 1987, the calendar was incorporated into the Magazine. Neither of these publications contain any record of the Club's activities or any members' ideas or concerns.

Club Members' Confidentiality

The organization in this study will be identified throughout this report as the "Club." A proper name will not be used as the Club requires confidentiality with regard to reports of group activities or identification of any individual member. The publication under study will be referred to as the "Magazine." Both reporting devices are used to try and conform to the Club members' desires for some secrecy about their often described "socially unacceptable" sexual expressions.

All material published in the Magazine is copyrighted by either the individual author or the Club. When a letter was received complaining that the Magazine had a copyright policy which was meant to protect the possible economic interests of the authors, the Club's Communication Secretary wrote, "In fact, we have an entirely different reason for copyrighting [the Magazine], and that has to do with the right of privacy of all our members."

Another example of confidentiality is the approval process necessary for using an audio or video recording device at a Club function. Prior approval for an electronic recording must be sought and granted during a Club business meeting, and all individuals appearing or heard on tape must sign a release which is then held in the Club's files. In addition, only clearly defined and marked spaces may be included in the video recording. Finally, all video equipment must have a real-time monitor separated from the camera's viewfinder so the recording process may be regulated by a Club officer.

The need for privacy seems to be an essential and overriding concern of the Club's members starting with new-member orientations. During this introductory process, potential new members must sign a form which states the person may not reveal the names and other identification information about other people at the orientations. All potential members are told they may be known by an assumed name, an S/M name, or simply by a first name. During this study, very few Club members used a full and real name for identification purposes.

Definitions

Some definitions will be helpful in understanding this report. A "scene" is an event in which two or more people engage in some type of "erotic power transference" for a predetermined period of time. The terms S/M (sadomasochism), B/D (bondage and discipline), and D/S (dominance and submission) will be used somewhat interchangeably. "Vanilla" is a term used to indicate heterosexual, middle-of-the-road, generally accepted sexual activity sanctioned by a majority of the general population and devoid of experimentation. The person engaged in a "scene" who is "in control" is called a "top," "master," or "mistress"; the person being controlled is termed a "bottom," "submissive," or "slave" (although, in fact, both actors are engaged in control, power transference, and the direction of the "scene").

Method

A descriptive content analysis by theme (Stempel and Westley 1981; Wimmer and Dominick 1986) was completed on forty-seven issues of the Magazine published by the Club between October 1983 and January 1988. The somewhat discontinuous nature of this monthly publication, which published forty-seven issues over a fifty-two-month period, is due to its dependence totally on a volunteer production staff. Utilizing descriptive categories, a numeric analysis was completed on the contents of the forty-seven issues. The results contain both percentages of the space allocated to subject categories and examples of the contents of those categories.

The December 1987 issue of the Magazine contained a twenty-six-question readership survey as a means of gathering information about the publication's future. The survey was initiated by the Club in response to internal organizational conflict between the two West Coast chapters. The January 1988 issue of the publication contained the survey results as 358 readers responded (representing 44% of the 812 dues-paying members). The survey results are used to support the content analysis.

As a supplement to the content analysis and the readership survey, this report includes information gathered by the author as a nonparticipant-observer of the Club's activities during the period covered by this study. The author attended a mandatory orientation session and approximately four program meetings each calendar year. The author discussed the Club and the Magazine with Club members during the orientation and programs.

Magazine Format

From October 1983 to January 1987, thirty-five issues of the Magazine were produced in a magazine format sized 7 inches by 8½ inches. In this format, the issues averaged 27.5 pages per issue, with a range of 22 pages to 46 pages. In February 1987, the Magazine's editor adopted a new format to allow for the easy use of desk-top publication computer software. The editor claimed the new format would be cost effective and would allow for a "more glitzy" publication. From February 1987 through January 1988, the format size changed to 8½ inches by 11 inches, the issues averaged sixteen pages, and the range was from eight to twenty pages. All issues were black ink on white paper stock.

Readership Survey Results

Almost the entire content of the January 1988 issue of the Magazine was dedicated to the results of the December 1987 readership survey. In addition to the survey question numeric results, ten of the publication's sixteen pages were filled with members' letters concerning the publication's future. In the letters, two major reasons were indicated as to why the survey was necessary: (a) The founding chapter produced the Magazine, all the Magazine's editors were from the founding chapter, and the other West Coast chapter's members complained the publication served little purpose to their interests; and (b) the publishing and mailing costs of the Magazine increased over time and some members questioned the ever-increasing expenditures.

The first seven questions of the readership survey were concerned with the Magazine's continuation and format. When asked if the Magazine should be eliminated, 10 readers marked "yes" and 339 marked "no." Four format questions elicited similar response patterns as the elimination question, with the vast majority of responses supporting the magazine format adopted in February 1987. The responses to cost questions were also favorable but more mixed. The founding chapter members responded positively by a 6 to 1 ratio when asked if $18 of the yearly $25 Club membership fee should be used to support the Magazine. The other West Coast chapter members were almost evenly divided on the fees question. When asked if the format should be changed to allow the magazine to fit in a 25-cent envelope, the founding chapter members marked "no" by a 6 to 1 ratio, while the other West Coast chapter members marked "no" by a 3 to 1 ratio. The ten pages of readers' letters included in the January 1988 issue indicated the writers were very strong in their support of the publication. The following statements came from several letters and reflected support sentiment:

> [The Magazine] should be recognized for what it is—the finest ongoing historical record of an S/M community ever compiled. . . . [The Club] will survive well without [the magazine], but its history will be lost forever. . . . An incredible and refreshing diversity of material has been presented. . . . [The Magazine] is an important erotic event in my life. . . . [The Magazine] is an important part of my membership. . . . It is a publication far superior to any other in the field. . . . Let's use this publication as a voice and a focal point.

"At-large" members, those living some distance from the Club's two chapters, also wrote in strong support of the publication:

I live in a foreign country [and] the whole [Club] to me is represented in the contents of [the Magazine]. . . . Thus [the Magazine] is my only tangible link to [the Club] and to the S/M community at large. . . . For individuals like me in extremely isolated areas, [the Magazine] is the only connection to the S/M world. . . . [The Magazine] is my sole connection to [the Club].

Content Analysis Results

The content analysis results of the forty-seven issues are reported under seven subject content areas: media reviews, poetry, S/M issues, how-to articles, photography, stories, and organizational reports. The seven areas are reported starting with the smallest amount of space utilized per category and continuing to the largest amount of space used.

Media Reviews

Reviews of books, films and videos with S/M themes appeared in about every second issue of the Magazine, averaged .5 items per issue, and accounted for about 2% of the space in the Magazine. Included in this category were reviews of S/M related story lines on "Hill Street Blues" (February 1986—all reference dates for materials from the Magazine refer to the publication date of that issue) and the "Oprah Winfrey Show" (August 1987), and the best location near the two Club chapters to purchase books, movies, and other S/M media materials. The readership respondents overwhelmingly indicated the media reviews category should be retained by a vote of 304 to 13.

Poetry

Poems appeared an average of 1.2 times per issue, with a range of no poems in several issues to six poems in one issue, and accounted for about 5% of the Magazine's space. Poems tended to concentrate on the feelings (both physical and emotional) expressed by a "top" or "bottom" with regard to a "scene." Several poems were written by "slaves" to their "masters" or "mistresses." The readership respondents indicated poems were the least favored content area with 139 votes for continuation, while 131 voted against continuation.

S/M Issues

Several types of S/M issue related articles appeared in the Magazine between 1983 and 1988. S/M issue articles and columns averaged 1.5 items per issue, ranged from a low of none in three issues to a high of six in two issues, and accounted for about 10% of the Magazine's space. Among the various discussions included in this category were long-term S/M relationships (June 1985), different levels of dominance (November 1985), masochistic "survival" (February 1985), a definition of torture (June 1985), and definitions of S/M terms (June 1985). One recurring interest area was the concept that D/S was a more inclusive term than S/M. As noted in an October/November 1984 article:

> D/S is a broader term inclusive of S/M just as both are included in a still broader category of 'creative sexuality.' While inclusive of S/M, D/S is not higher or better than S/M. On the contrary, S/M is a special (some feel 'elite') subgroup within the broader context of D/S.

In July 1985 another writer agreed to the ideas expressed in the October/November 1984 article and added: "D/S doesn't have to be physically rough, nor does it require pain, fetishes—or even sex!"

Legal action against people engaged in S/M activities were reported. Information about a Sacramento, California, professional dominant who had been arrested for prostitution was included in issues starting with October 1983 and running until the middle of 1985. The cases of a Pennsylvania couple and a Michigan couple who ran into problems with the legal authorities were included in 1985 and 1986.

When asked about reporting legal actions, 289 respondents marked "yes," while 22 respondents marked "no." The readers also responded they wanted "reprints of S/M materials from nonmembers" by a 244 to 37 margin, and they responded with 280 "yes" and 18 "no" when asked about inclusion of "clippings of relevant S/M materials."

How-to Information

How-to information appeared in virtually every issue. This category averaged 2.4 items per issue, ranged from no items in one issue to seven items in six issues, and took up about 12% of the Magazine's space. How-to article titles indicated the subject matter including: "Building Clothes Pins with a Screw Device" (October/November 1983) for attaching to a "bottom's" body, "Fur Braiding" (January 1985) for braiding rope in pubic hair, and "An Example of a Slavery Contract" (November 1986). In the how-to category, safety and health issues received a great deal of attention. Health problems related to AIDS received the most attention.

A readership survey question asking if how-to articles and "doing S/M" articles should be included received an overwhelmingly positive response with 320 readers marking "yes" and 15 respondents marking "no."

Photography

Over the forty-seven issues which were content analyzed, the average was 7.5 photographs per issue, the range was no photographs in nine issues to thirty-nine photographs in the October/November 1984 issues, and these images accounted for 14% of the Magazine's space. The photographs were primarily of erotic images by members and of local and national S/M events.

Accounting for almost half of all photographs, erotic images included one or more individuals tied in tight bondage with various devices attached to their bodies. Other photographs included both the "top" and the "bottom" at play in either private or public settings. Facial expressions ranged from the exhibitionist who seemed pleased that his or her picture was being taken, to the grimaces of "bottoms" who were in some type of painful scene. Results of the readership survey indicated members wanted "erotic photographs by members" by a rate of 283 "yes" to 23 "no," and "photos of local or national S/M events" by a margin of 229 "yes" to 52 "no."

Stories

Stories, both real and fantasy, averaged 1.5 per issue, ranged from no stories in five issues to three stories in three issues, and accounted for 17% of the Magazine's space.

Fantasy stories tended to fall into those with "vanilla" titles and those with very explicit titles. The first group included stories titled "Wednesday Afternoon" (May 1985) and "The Plan" (May 1987). More explicit titles included "Nocturnal Emissions from a Submissive" (August 1984) and "Scat 'n Shower Delights" (October 1987) focusing on scatological and "golden shower" interests.

Stories of real scenes tended to be forthright in their titles, subject matter, and accompanying photographs. One real column, titled "A Slave Girl Writes," was included in five 1985 issues and was written by female "slaves." "Viola's Slave Diary" was included in the October through December 1987 issues. As noted earlier, all the stories were copyrighted with 93% including an author's name and 7% indicating the Club held the copyright.

"Erotic fiction" should be included by a vote of the readers of 297 to 25, and "real-life S/M experiences" should be continued by a response of 297 "yes" to 25 "no."

Organization

The largest content category, both in terms of space and number of items, was devoted to Club organizational activities. Organizational items accounted for an average of 6.5 items per issue, ranged from three items in four issues to twelve items in nine issues, and accounted for 40% of the Magazine's space.

Among the most common organization reports were: Complete monthly statements from the Club's treasurer, a column from the editor, reports from the Club's coordinator(s), membership reports, and extensive reports from the Communication Secretary (July 1984 to November 1987) or "Comm Sexy" as the column was signed.

A column titled the "Slave Trader's Marketplace" was included in each issue. Professional "play for pay" advertisements were not allowed because it was felt this type of advertising would bring the magazine and the organization to the attention of law enforcement agencies.

The Magazine reported on Club sponsored meetings. Approximately two theme programs were presented by the Club each month during the period of this study. The subjects of these programs, presented in the Magazine's coverage, included: an ask-a-lawyer discussion (October/November 1984), a flagellation discussion/demonstration (December 1984), a founders' panel (February 1985), a body piercing demonstration (October/November 1984), a use of electricity demonstration (December 1985), an ask-a-chiropractor discussion (January 1987), a male genital torture discussion/demonstration (April 1987), and various panels by and about dominance and submission (March 1985, July 1985, and August/September 1985).

Several readership survey questions asked about organizational presentations in the Magazine. When asked if the readers wanted to read about "local club events and programs," 296 marked "yes" and 22 marked "no." When asked about the inclusion of the "Treasurer's reports and other club business reports," the respondents marked "yes" 171 times and "no" was checked by 86 readers. Even "classified or display advertising" should be kept in the Magazine according to 295 respondents who marked "yes" as opposed to the 12 readers who marked "no."

The seven subject categories outlined in these results include virtually all the material published in the Magazine from 1983 through early 1988 (which indicates that the content analysis categories were exhaustive). In the 47 issues which were investigated, the Club's activities and organizational information accounted for almost one-half of all publication space. Additionally, in descending order of the publication's space utilization, stories accounted for 17%, photography accounted for 14%, how-to information accounted for 12%, S/M issues accounted for about 2%.

The readership survey results published in the January 1988 issue indicate the respondents want to keep all the subject categories. While poetry received almost an even split vote, all the other subject areas received enthusiastic support from the survey respondents. The results indicate the Club members wish to continue the Magazine with 358 respondents (representing 44% of the total Club membership) responding positively by almost a 20 to 1 ratio.

Editors

All four of the Magazine's editors who worked during this study called for contributions to the Magazine by the Club's members, and they all stressed the participatory nature of the publication. One editor called in June 1985 for more members' input and then promised to "remain aware of the printed word's iconic powers and to remain sensitive to members' feelings." Another editor called in April 1987 for material which was not mediocre but was "brought to life by being handled with verve, originality, and some skill." The problem, that editor continued, was trite storylines and "doggerel" poetry that tended to make the contributions less interesting.

One editor indicated in October 1986 his editorial stance by writing that the Magazine was a tool for communicating. In a particularly lucid moment, this editor wrote about the worth of the publication:

> [The Magazine] brings the membership an arena of common experience and concern. Each month of appearance is evidence of our energy and our pride—and our power. Because it is controlled by us, [the Magazine] can tell the evolving truth: no advertisers, governmental agencies, or professional practitioners! . . . We know the feelings of guilt, bewilderment, and isolation; we also know freedom and happiness when we can admit, discuss and demonstrate those feelings. [The Club] and [the Magazine], if you will, smooth a few steps on the road to happiness.

This editor went on to explain the publication operates as the only legacy and historical document of the organization, and about half of the yearly dues go into the support of the publication.

Discussion

The results of this study indicate that the Magazine is a creation of the Club's membership and that membership is satisfied with the publication's format and contents. The January 1988 readership study and the content analysis results point toward strong support for the publication's place in the lives of the Club members.

In addition to being the only repository of the Club's history and the importance of the Magazine to individual members, the publication may serve to help create "shared meaning" for Club members. Researchers Berger and Luckman (1967) argue that a social institution "can only be understood in terms of the 'knowledge' that its members have of it, [and] it follows that the analysis of such 'knowledge' will be essential for an analysis of the institution in question" (p. 65). These writers further assert that once the body of social knowledge is given meaning by the collective understanding of the group, that meaning "has the capacity to act back upon the collectivity that produced it" (p. 85). As stated by one Magazine editor, "Through [the Magazine], we share experiences which few people in the world understand, and develop new vocabulary and concepts. Shared, our experiences become a legacy for every newcomer" (October 1986). The Magazine's editors and readers seem to agree that the publication is vital and provides opportunities to explain and explore their sadomasochistic experiences.

The "shared" experiences of Club members which is chronicled in the Magazine is a legacy to increasing numbers of Club members. During the period of this investigation, October 1983 to January 1988, the Club's membership increased by over 400%. The change in membership was of type as well as number. During the author's discussions with long-time members and through the author's nonparticipant observations of the audience composition for Club programs, the Club's membership was primarily male homosexuals at the end of 1983. Indeed, members' comments indicated male gays comprised virtually the entire membership between the Club's founding in 1974 and the early 1980s. From 1983 to 1988 a dramatic increase of both gay and heterosexual women was witnessed at program meetings. Male-female couples were at the end of this study about one-third of all participants at program meetings. By the start of 1988, a majority of the Club members were heterosexual men, women, and couples; of course, many members were still homosexual men and women. The approach taken in this study is not appropriate to explicate the changes brought about by the changes in the makeup of the membership of the Club; however, the demographic changes are interesting and would provide the basis for a future study.

An issue highlighted through this research concerns the forces acting on an organization dedicated to alternative sexual practices. Contained in the Club's purpose statement is that the organization should attempt to help the public understand the S/M subcultures. Yet access to the Club and its Magazine is restricted. Only dues-paying Club members receive the publication, copyright and confidentiality statements are prominent in the Magazine, entrance into programs and meetings is granted to card-carrying members and their guests only, and most members use either an S/M "name" or are called by their first names.

Personal questions about a member's employment and residence, even in the most general terms, are greeted with some suspicion. The call for public education is clearly restrained by the need for individual members to retain some measure of privacy as a means of escaping scorn.

The duality of public knowledge versus the private rights expressed in the Magazine reflects the conflicting forces of the larger society with respect to sexual expression. Respondents to a 1987 Associated Press poll thought pornography was not generally harmful to adults, 80% admitted to having looked at and enjoyed a magazine featuring nudity, and 60% had seen an X-rated movie on video cassette ("Poll says most Americans unoffended by pornography," 1987). The newspaper article which outlined the poll findings also pointed out the war on "smut" launched by U.S. Attorney General Edwin Meese and the increasing number of attempts to ban magazines such as *Playboy* from retail store shelves. What the people of the United States may like and practice in private does not seem to be acceptable when expressed or available in public.

The emergence of social science research on sadomasochistic activities which is just now appearing (Weinberg 1987) may be due, in part, to the muting of emotions raised by the study of so-called "deviant" individuals that has plagued social science researchers in the past. Even now the way is not clear and unprejudiced. Many of the highly educated and sophisticated people the author encountered during this research were embarrassed or otherwise incapable of discussing the subject matter.

Summary

The research reported here is broadly descriptive in nature. Focusing on the activities of a sadomasochism Club as detailed in the pages of the Club's magazine, this study combined a readership survey and a subject content analysis to reveal: (a) The Magazine is the Club's only record, (b) the publication is a legacy for new Club members and others interested in this S/M sub-culture, and (c) the Magazine is the codification of "shared" meanings created by Club members.

The major weakness of this investigation is the lack of actor viewpoint data. As noted by Berger and Luckman (1967), a group's participants create their shared realities. In addition, sadomasochism subcultures are, by necessity, somewhat secre-tive. For those reasons, the participants' viewpoint is necessary in understanding the subculture. Despite the inclusion of the author's nonparticipant observations, this study lacks under-standing from the actor's point of view. Future research could concentrate on the members' communication strategies as a means of understanding the creation of group-shared meanings. The interpersonal power negotiations utilized by S/M interest-ed people is also a fertile area of future study. Utilizing qualita-tive data gathering methods, the "secret" S/M groups could be better understood. Value-free approaches must be used or the researcher will fall victim to the negative opinions concerning "deviant" sexual expressions held by the society at large.

This study does suggest that this type of magazine and other "house organs" of S/M groups are sources for understanding the activities of group members. It would seem that this Maga-zine, for the members of this Club, is truly a "tie that binds."

Note

The term "Club" was selected to identify the organization as many club-like attributes have been adopted by the organization under investigation. A prospective member must be eighteen years of age, must pay a fee to join and a fee to continue yearly membership. S/he must be issued and use a membership identification card to gain entry to Club activities. If the prospective member lives within an hour's drive of either of the two West Coast chapters, s/he is required to attend a "mandatory" orientation.

References

Berger, P. L., and T. Luckman. 1967. *The Social Construction of Reality.* Garden City, N.Y.: Doubleday.

Breslow, B., L. Evans, and J. Langley. 1985. "On the Prevalence and Roles of Females in the Sadomasochistic Subculture: Report of an Empirical Study." *Archives of Sexual Behavior* 14 (4): 303–17.

————. (1986). "Comparisons among Heterosexual, Bisexual, and Homosexual Male Sado-masochists." *Journal of Homosexuality* 13 (1): 83–107.

Naerseen, A. X., van, M. van Dijk, G. Hoogveen, and G. van Zessen. 1987. "Gay SM in Pornography and Reality." *Journal of Homosexuality* 12 (2/3): 111–19.

"Poll Says Most Americans Unoffended by Pornography." 1987. *The Stockton Record* (April 12), p. A–7.

Stempel, G. H., and B. H. Westley, eds. 1981. *Research Methods in Mass Communication.* Englewood Cliffs, N.J.: Prentice-Hall.

Weinberg, T. S. 1987. "Sadomasochism in the United States: A Review of Recent Sociological Literature." *The Journal of Sex Research* 23 (1): 50–69.

Wimmer, R. D., and J. R. Dominick. 1986. *Mass Media Research: An Introduction.* Belmont, Calif.: Wadsworth.

SYNTHESIS
DEVELOPING A SEXOLOGY
OF SADOMASOCHISM

Thomas S. Weinberg

Sociological and Social Psychological Issues in the Study of Sadomasochism

Several years ago I published a review of the sociological literature on sadomasochism (Weinberg 1987). While there have been a number of important contributions to the study of this topic since that time, they have all reinforced my original perspective, that S&M is most realistically viewed as a social behavior. This sociological point of view is supported by other writers who have broadened the earlier psychoanalytic approach of, for example, Freud (1905/1953, 1920/1961, 1924/1959), Krafft-Ebing (1886/1965), and Stekel (1929/1965), who viewed sadomasochism as evidence of individual psychopathology. These more modern writers reflect a unifying theme pioneered by Gebhard (1969) and developed by others beginning in the late 1970s (e.g., Falk and Weinberg 1983; Kamel 1980, 1983a, 1983b; Lee 1979; Moser 1979; Patrias 1978; Scott 1983; Scoville 1984; Spengler 1977, 1979; Weinberg 1978; Weinberg and Falk 1980; Weinberg and Kamel 1983; M. Weinberg, Williams, and Moser 1984) that S&M is dependent upon meanings, which

Reprinted from Thomas S. Weinberg, "Research in Sadomasochism: A Review of Sociological and Social Psychological Literature," *Annual Review of Sex Research* 1994, vol. 5: 257–79. Reprinted by permission of the publisher and the author.

are culturally produced, learned, and reinforced by participation in the sadomasochistic subculture.

With an accumulation of almost two decades of research on and theorizing about sadomasochism from the sociological and social psychological perspectives, we are now at a point where some consensus has developed on a number of issues. The first task in the study of S&M is to define it. This would appear at first to be difficult because, as many writers have noted, the behaviors and identities within the sadomasochistic subculture are tremendously varied. It is certainly true that there are a variety of S&M worlds; and there is tremendous diversity among groups as well as individuals in terms of their preferences and tastes (e.g., bondage, transvestism, verbal humiliation, enemas, urination, feces, whips, a wide range of interest in and tolerance of pain). However, there are commonalities that override distinctions of sexual orientation and specific behaviors. Falk and I (Falk and Weinberg 1983) have noted a few essential characteristics of the current American S&M scene: It is erotic, consensual, and recreational. As recreational or play-like behavior, it involves fantasy in varying degrees (Brodsky 1993), which, in turn, requires some collaboration to carry out satisfactorily (Baumeister 1988b; Weinberg 1978; Weinberg and Falk 1980). Additionally, M. Weinberg et al. (1984) have observed that the situation must be mutually defined by all participants as both sexual and S&M. This last idea requires that participants "frame" their behavior in certain ways (Goffman 1974; Lee 1979; Weinberg 1978) by the use of social definitions that give the behavior a specific contextual meaning.

Symbolic interactionist and phenomenological approaches tell us that if we wish to understand S&M motivations and behavior, we must look to the definitions provided by these people rather than attempt to impose our own preconceived notions upon this activity (Moser 1979; M. Weinberg et al. 1984). Failure to view S&M behavior and motivations within its social context risks "misframing" (Goffman 1974) and thus misinterpreting what is going on (Moser 1984).

Pain

Pain has traditionally been subsumed in definitions of sado-masochism (Ellis 1903/1926; Freud 1905/1953; Gebhard 1969; Spengler 1977). Breslow (1989) and Moser (1988) include both psychological and physical pain in their definitions. However, despite the attempt of some writers to emphasize the importance of pain to sadomasochists, it is not, as Gebhard (1969) pointed out, necessarily perceived by S&M practitioners *themselves* as central to or even necessary for S&M. Baumeister (1988a) noted that "pain is not universal in masochistic experiences" (p. 37) and when it occurs it "seem(s) to be carefully limited" (ibid.). Myers (1992) pointed out that "SM does not have to involve pain. There are many people who prefer a gentler approach to what otherwise would be considered SM" (p. 302). Moser and Levitt (1987) noted problems in using pain as part of the definition of S&M. They are "(a) the pain experience itself is altered during sexual arousal, (b) not all pain is arousing to avowed sadomasochists, and (c) some S/M experiences (e.g., restraint) are not painful" (p. 322). Both Spengler (1977) and Moser (1979) found that "the extreme and dangerous S/M practices recurred with a minimal frequency" (Moser 1979, p. 54), and Moser further indicated that most of his respondents were involved in, enjoyed most, and believed their partners most enjoyed, "medium" S&M interaction. Houlberg (1991) quotes an S&Mer, who writes that this behavior "doesn't have to be physically rough, nor does it require pain, fetishes—or even sex!" (p. 175). Califia, herself a practitioner, felt that, "The basic dynamic of S&M is the power dichotomy, not pain" (Califia 1979, p. 21). Similarly, Kamel and I, commenting on the variety of nonpainful acts preferred by many S&Mers, have noted that, "It is the illusion of violence, rather than violence itself, that is frequently arousing to both sadists and masochists. At the very core of sadomasochism is not pain but the idea of control—dominance and submission" (Weinberg and Kamel 1983, p. 20).

    Pain, then, does not appear to be necessary to S&M. However, it does appear in many S&M scenarios. The question then becomes, what is its function? A number of answers to this question have been proposed. Ellis (1903/1926) pointed out that pain can serve as a sexual stimulant. Gebhard (1969) also emphasized the arousal properties of pain, while being careful to point out that pain has many meanings for sadomasochists. Mass (1979) speculated that pain can trigger the production of endorphins, which may result in a feeling of euphoria and well-being. Baumeister (1988a) believed that the function of pain for S&Mers may be "as a technique for removing higher-level self-awareness, while promoting a low-level awareness of self as physical object. Pain brings self-awareness down from symbolic identity to physical body" (p. 39). A more sociological explanation for the presence of pain in some sadomasochistic situations is provided by M. Weinberg et al. (1984). They noted that pain is often used to express dominance and submission. This may, in fact, be its primary appeal for some S&Mers. It may not be pain itself, but what it *symbolizes* (i.e., that one is completely in control of or under the control of, another person) that is erotic for some people. Moser (1988) explains that "both physical and psychological behaviors are devised to emphasize the transfer of power from the submissive to the dominant partner. S/M practitioners often report it is this consentual (sic) exchange of power that is erotic to them and the pain is just a method of achieving this power exchange" (p. 50). It is not my intention to deny the importance of pain to *some* S&M practitioners nor to ignore the possibility that pain can be eroticized, but to point out that definitions that focus exclusively on pain miss the essence of S&M, the ritualization of dominance and submission. These definitions, therefore, ignore the complexity of S&M. It is rich in symbolism and heavily dependent upon shared meanings, which are learned within the subculture and which serve to structure S&M interaction.

Dominance and Submission

The key to understanding S&M as a social phenomenon, as a number of writers have pointed out (Califia 1979; Gebhard 1969; Kamel 1983b; Scott 1983; Scoville 1984; Weinberg and Kamel 1983; M. Weinberg et al. 1984), is to view it in terms of patterns of dominance and submission. In emphasizing this point, both Scott (1983) and Scoville (1984) used the expression D/S (dominance and submission) to refer to the heterosexual S&M scene. Houlberg (1991) used the terms S/M, D/S, and B/D (bondage and discipline) interchangeably. He noted that sadomasochistic practitioners see D/S as a broader term that includes S&M. There is, however, a difference of opinion on the theme underlying dominance and submission. Some writers see the issue of *control* as central (e.g., Weinberg and Kamel 1983), whereas others (e.g., Myers 1992; Scoville 1984) emphasize *trust*. Both M. Weinberg et al. (1984) and I (Weinberg 1978) have underscored the *fantasy* element involved in dominance and submission. It would appear to be most accurate to include all three elements in a discussion of S&M, though not necessarily in the same degree.

While ideas of self as dominant or submissive appear to be important to some participants in the S&M scene, a number of writers have found that a sizeable proportion of people in the scene are "flexible" or "switchable" in role choice (Breslow et al. 1985; Califia 1979; Gebhard 1969; Kamel 1980; Kamel and Weinberg 1983; Moser 1988; Moser and Levitt 1987; Naerssen et al. 1987; Spengler 1977; Weinberg 1978). Thus, it would seem that for many people it is the behavior or scene that is critical, not one's specific role in it (Kamel and Weinberg 1983).

Limits, Fantasy, and Control

The issues of limits, fantasy, and control are intertwined, and all of them are related in one way or another to the issue of trust. One of the questions addressed by researchers, theorists, and practitioners of S&M is whether the dominant or the submissive has the control in an S&M scenario. While some practitioners feel that the submissive should be able to control the interaction because neither partner could precisely know what his limits are beforehand (Naerssen et al. 1987), this does not appear to be an accurate description of what usually happens during a scene. Probably the most realistic description of what actually occurs is that both dominants and submissives are actively involved in the development of the scenario (Califia 1979; Kamel 1980; Kamel and Weinberg 1983; Lee 1979). In an S&M scene, the action is often, but not always, scripted and therefore collaborative, so that neither the dominant nor the submissive usually has complete control.

Although limits are usually discussed by practitioners who do not know each other well, prior to engaging in S&M, this does not mean that they are rigidly adhered to as the scene unfolds. Limit setting and scripting vary widely from the most casual to the very elaborate (Lee 1979), so that some situations leave a great deal of room for innovation. In addition, the scenario is an interactive situation that evolves differently each time, so that what occurs is partly the result of the ways in which the responses of each partner are interpreted and responded to by the other. Essentially, the limits are "determined during the game" (Naerssen et al. 1987, p. 118). Often, signals used to control the interaction are nonverbal and very subtle. A scene often requires a great deal of trust in the alertness and sensitivity of the dominant. For example, I observed the following interaction in Paddles, an S&M club in New York City:

> When we walked into the club, a scene was already underway. A man in his thirties was lying on his back, secured to a table with leather straps. His legs, genitals, chest, and upper arms were bound with a ribbon of thin black leather. Only his lower arms, from the elbows down, and hands were free. A dominant dressed in black leather was whipping his legs with a cock whip, a small cat-o-nine-tails about a foot long. She was moving the whip slowly, drawing it along his legs with each stroke.

> She was using her elbows, not swinging from the shoulder or snapping the whip with her wrist. She struck his testicles, and he started. Very slowly, without saying anything, he moved his hands up and cupped his genitals. Without a word, the dominatrix gently removed his hands, unwrapped his penis and testicles, wrapped his forearms, and slowly shifted her whip to his chest.

Many S&M scenes contain at least a fictive (i.e., fantasy) control element (Kamel 1980; Magill 1982). Within the fantasy frame, participants attempt to maintain an illusion of reality. During the transition into a scene, adjustments are made subtly, to maintain the fiction that the submissive is dependent upon the will of the dominant:

> Three dominant women were preparing a submissive for a scene. They tied his legs together, threw the free end of the rope over a hook in the wall about six feet off the ground, and began to hoist him up by the legs, while his upper body was resting on a table. Two of the women asked him in a barely audible whisper whether he was uncomfortable. He nodded to assure them that he was okay.

It is possible that limits are determined as much by the evolving fantasy as they are by physiological considerations, such as pain thresholds. Another hypothesis for testing involves the clarity and detail with which scripts are elaborated and limits are set. This may vary with the degree of intimacy, so that those situations in which intimacy is greatest, such as interaction with a lover, who knows one's needs, tend to be loosely defined, whereas scenarios with strangers tend to be more closely controlled. Frequent interaction should lessen the need for specific guidelines, not only because of increasing familiarity, but also because of the development of trust.

Trust is an important theme for S&Mers. Myers (1992) observed two types of burning engaged in by S&M nonmainstream body modifiers. One of these, "play burning," "capitalizes on the classic SM goals of trust and the *threat* (italics in original) of pain and/or injury, but does so without leaving intentional burn marks" (p. 304). Trust inheres not just in the relationship established between the partners, but may also be built into the structure of the S&M subculture, especially when the actors are relative strangers. Some writers have noted that a concern with one's reputation within the subculture and the recognition that this may affect the consequent availability of partners may serve to keep behavior within acceptable bounds (Lee 1979; M. Weinberg et al. 1984). Related to trust is the issue of safety, both in terms of the reliability of one's partner (Lee 1979) and in practices and equipment (Houlberg 1991; Myers 1992).

Identity

One area in which there is little information is that of the acquisition of and commitment to S&M identities. There are two separate issues here: the etiology of an S&M desire or preference and the translation of these needs by the individual into a particular identity. Psychodynamic theories that attempt to explain the development of sadomasochistic desires are quite distinct from sociological explanations of the process by which people come to realize these needs, find other people with whom to act them out, and develop an idea of self as "dominant" ("top," "Master," "Mistress") or "submissive" ("bottom," "slave").

Some preliminary sociological research seems to indicate that psychodynamic theories may not be relevant to the identity development of many S&M practitioners (Breslow 1989). For example, Moser and Levitt (1987) found that only 18.6% of their sample recalled having received erotic enjoyment from being punished as a child. Moser concluded that, "the results do not support or negate a developmental etiology for the behavior" (1979, p. 75). Breslow et al. (1986) found that only 5.4% of their sample felt that they had been sexually abused as children, and just slightly more than one-fourth claimed to have been emotionally abused. M. Weinberg et al. (1984) do not deny that the traditional medical model "accurately represents some people," but they argue, as Kamel and I have done (Weinberg and Kamel 1983), that "such a viewpoint does not do justice to the majority of persons and phenomena to which the label `sadomasochism' is applied" (M. Weinberg et al. 1984, p. 380). It would be premature, however, to discount the importance of psychodynamic theories in the etiology of sadomasochism, for at least some S&Mers, on the basis of what are still unconfirmed findings.

Patrias (1978) and Kamel and I (Kamel and Weinberg 1983) point out that the development of an S&M identity is part of an interactive process; that is, a "career." Those who have recognized their sadomasochistic feelings and desires must seek out others who share them. Then they must learn to construct and control S&M scenarios. Through socialization they learn specific norms and values. Integration into the S&M subculture appears to be positively correlated with adjustment to self-identity as an S&Mer. Spengler found "a number of significant correlations which indicate that subcultural integration (defined by the frequency of participation in sadomasochistic parties) and the possibility of realizing the deviance in a partnership context are associated with self-acceptance" (Spengler 1977, p. 450). Breslow et al. (1985, 1986) and Moser and Levitt (1987) also found a high degree of self-acceptance among S&Mers.

Some people, who have not previously recognized any sadomasochistic interests, become involved in S&M through a variety of relationships. For example, women married to men with interests in dominance and submission may eventually be induced to participate in S&M and even come to enjoy it (Kamel and Weinberg 1983). Over 60 percent of the women in the Breslow et al. (1985) study had been introduced to S&M by another person. Certainly, more research is needed both on the genesis of certain desires and identities and on the processes by which they come to be realized.

Additional Directions for Further Research

There is still not enough theory building and empirical research in S&M. Few theoretical papers in sociology and social psychology have been published, and they have been very narrowly focused. Only a handful of surveys of samples of sadomasochists have been done, and they are over ten years old (Breslow et al. 1985, 1986; Moser 1979; Spengler 1977). Additionally, more field research, collecting observational and interview data, guided by theoretical frameworks, is necessary.

We are still in an early stage of knowledge about S&M, with little or no information about a number of topics. An important question that has been ignored is that of how the AIDS crisis has affected the S&M community. The literature has been silent about this. Only Houlberg (1991) mentioned in passing that "the health problems related to AIDS have received the most attention" (p. 176) in the sadomasochistic magazine he analyzed. It is quite possible that S&M has become a popular substitute for genital sex among some groups. For some sadomasochists, a genital orgasm is not necessary during an S&M scene (Naerssen et al. 1987). S&Mers often talk about "whether a particular body modification or play technique would produce a genital orgasm or an equal thrill in the mind ('head orgasm') or both" (Myers 1992, p. 304). Within the sadomasochistic community, one wonders, if there has been a switch from, for example, practices that may cause bleeding to nonintrusive behaviors such as spanking or verbal humiliation.

One important area for research is the S&M relationship. Scoville (1984) claims that there are "precious few ongoing live-in relationships" (p. 33) between S&M people and that "since there are no societal supports, domination relationships, where they exist, are usually of short duration" (p. 35). Breslow et al. (1986) noted that large proportions of heterosexuals and bisexuals in their study had a significant other with whom they were open about their S&M sexual interests. No indication is given, however, of how many of these respondents engaged in S&M

regularly with these significant others. Moser (1988) and Myers (1992) noted the presence of S&M couples.

Symbolism is a strong element in the S&M subculture. Within that world, certain elements, such as, for example, particular articles of clothing, take on special meanings, which are culturally produced, learned, and reinforced. This symbolism is illustrated in S&M magazines, which picture S&M participants in standardized costumes, most often in leather or rubber garments. Women are often clothed in tight corsets, garter belts, and high boots. The meaning of this apparel for participants in the S&M subculture has not yet been explored, although there is an apparent consensus within that community that goes beyond its special significance for the individual. There is a need to investigate the possible relationships between personal symbolism and culturally reinforced motifs within the S&M world.

Conclusions

Although individuals and S&M sex scenes have received some attention, little interest has been paid to the social conditions producing this behavior. If the focus of research is shifted from the individual to the larger society, the basic question, "Why do some people become 'sadomasochistic'?" is thus transformed, more sociologically, to "What are the social conditions under which S&M occurs in a society?" Another way of putting this is, "what is there about certain societies that encourages or allows this mode of erotic expression?" Gebhard (1969) addressed this very question. He claimed that sadomasochism (as a *social* phenomenon) is found only in well-developed civilizations. Although he acknowledged that biting and scratching may be found as part of sexual behavior in preliterate societies, "well-developed sadomasochism as a lifestyle is conspicuous by its absence" (Gebhard 1969, p. 80). He hypothesized that, "It may be that a society must be extremely complex and heavily reliant upon symbolism before the inescapable repressions and frustrations of life in such a society can be expressed symbolically in sadomasochism" (Gebhard 1969, p. 80). Baumeister's (1988a) thesis of masochism makes a similar assumption that modern pressures and responsibilities may become burdensome, motivating individuals to escape from self.

We get some additional clues bearing upon the areas to explore in seeking an answer to this question by looking at the critical features of S&M: It is erotic, consensual, and recreational. It is heavily dependent upon fantasy and the illusion of control, and it requires collaboration and mutual definitions in order to be satisfying to the participants.

It might be hypothesized based on the preceding discussion, that individual sadomasochistic interests become institutionalized into an S&M subculture in societies that fill the following criteria: (a) dominance-submission relationships are embedded in the culture and aggression is socially valued (Gebhard 1969); (b) there is a well developed and unequal distribution of power between social categories (e.g., the sexes, social classes, etc.), which may make the temporary illusion of its reversal erotically stimulating (Kamel 1980; Lee 1979; Weinberg 1978); (c) there is sufficient affluence enjoyed by at least some segments of the population to enable them to experience leisure-time activities (Falk and Weinberg 1983); and (d) imagination and creativity are encouraged and valued assets, as evidenced by the importance of scripts and fantasy in S&M (Lee 1979; M. Weinberg et al. 1984; Weinberg 1978).

References

Baumeister, R. F. 1988a. "Masochism as Escape from Self." *Journal of Sex Research* 25: 28–59.

———. 1988b. "Gender Differences in Masochistic Scripts." *Journal of Sex Research* 25: 478–99.

Breslow, N. 1987. "Locus of Control, Desirability of Control, and Sado-masochists." *Psychological Reports* 61: 995–1001.

Breslow, N. 1989. "Sources of Confusion in the Study and Treatment of Sadomasochism." *Journal of Social Behavior and Personality* 4: 263–74.

Breslow, N., L. Evans, and J. Langley. 1985. "On the Prevalence and Roles of Females in the Sadomasochistic Subculture: Report of an Empirical Study." *Archives of Sexual Behavior* 14: 303–17.

———. 1986. "Comparisons among Heterosexual, Bisexual, and Homosexual Male Sadomasochists." *Journal of Homosexuality* 13 (1): 83–107.

Brodsky, J. I. 1993."The Mineshaft: A Retrospective Ethnography." *Journal of Homosexuality* 24 (3/4): 233–51.

Califia, P. 1979. "A Secret Side of Lesbian Sexuality." *The Advocate* (December 17): 19–23.

Ellis, H. 1926. *Studies in the Psychology of Sex, Vol. 3, Analysis of the Sexual Impulse, Love and Pain, the Sexual Impulse in Women*, 2d ed., revised and enlarged. Philadelphia: F. A. Davis. (Original work published in 1903)

Falk, G., and T. S. Weinberg. 1983. "Sadomasochism and Popular Western Culture," in *S&M: Studies in Sadomasochism*, ed. T. Weinberg & G. W. L. Kamel, pp. 137–44. Amherst, N.Y.: Prometheus Books.

Freud, S. 1953. "Three Essays on Sexuality," in *The Standard Edition of the Complete Psychological Works of Sigmund Freud*, vol. 7, ed. and trans. J. Strachey, pp. 135–230. London: Hogarth Press. (Original work published in 1905)

———. 1959."The Economic Problem in Masochism," in *Sigmund Freud, Collected Papers*, ed. E. Jones, trans. J. Riviere, vol. 2, pp. 255–76. New York: Basic Books. (Original work published in 1924)

———. 1961. *Beyond the Pleasure Principle*, ed. and trans. J. Strachey. New York: Liveright. (Original work published in 1920)

Gebhard, P. 1969. "Fetishism and Sadomasochism," in *Dynamics of Deviant Sexuality*, ed. J. H. Masserman, pp. 71–80. New York: Grune & Stratton.

Goffman, E. 1974. *Frame Analysis*. Cambridge, Mass.: Harvard University Press.

Houlberg, R. 1991. "The Magazine of a Sadomasochistic Club: The Tie that Binds." *Journal of Homosexuality* 21 (1/2): 167–83.

Innala, S. M., and K. E. Ernulf. 1992. "Understanding Male Homosexual Attraction: An Analysis of Restroom Graffiti." *Journal of Social Behavior and Personality* 7: 503–10.

Kamel, G. W. L. 1980. "Leathersex: Meaningful Aspects of Gay Sadomasochism." *Deviant Behavior: An Interdisciplinary Journal* 1: 171–91.

———. 1983a. "The Leather Career: On Becoming a Sadomasochist," In *S&M: Studies in Sadomasochism*, ed. T. Weinberg and G. W. L. Kamel, pp. 73–79. Amherst, N.Y.: Prometheus Books.

———. 1983b. "Toward a Sexology of Sadomasochism," in *S&M: Studies in Sadomasochism*, ed. T. Weinberg and G. W. L. Kamel, pp. 197–203. Amherst, N.Y.: Prometheus Books.

Kamel, G. W. L., and T. S. Weinberg. 1983. "Diversity in Sadomasochism: Four S&M Careers," in *S&M: Studies in Sadomasochism*, ed. T. Weinberg & G. W. L. Kamel, pp. 113–28. Amherst, N.Y.: Prometheus Books.

Krafft-Ebing, R. V. 1965. *Psychopathia Sexualis,* trans. F. S. Klaf. New York: Stein & Day. (Original work published in 1886)

Lee, J. A. 1979. "The Social Organization of Sexual Risk." *Alternative Lifestyles* 2: 69–100.

Magill, M. S. 1982. *Ritual and Symbolism of Dominance and Submission: The Case of Heterosexual Sadomasochism.* State University of New York at Buffalo. (Unpublished manuscript)

Mass, L. 1979. "Coming to Grips with Sadomasochism." *The Advocate,* (April 5): 18–22.

Moser, C. 1979. *An Exploratory-descriptive Study of a Self-defined S/M (Sadomasochistic) Sample.* Institute for Advanced Study of Human Sexuality, San Francisco, Calif. (Unpublished manuscript)

———. 1984. "*Dominant women-submissive men: An exploration in erotic dominance and submission*" [Book review]. *The Journal of Sex Research* 20: 417–19.

———. 1988. "Sadomasochism." *Journal of Social Work and Human Sexuality* 7 (1): 43–56.

Moser, C., and E. E. Levitt. 1987. "An Exploratory-descriptive Study of a Sadomasochistically Oriented Sample." *Journal of Sex Research* 23: 322–37.

Myers, J. 1992. "Nonmainstream Body Modification: Genital Piercing, Branding, Burning, and Cutting." *Journal of Contemporary Ethnography* 21: 267–306.

Naerseen, A. X. van, M. van Dijk, G. Hoogveen, and G. van Zessen. 1987. "Gay SM in Pornography and Reality." *Journal of Homosexuality,* 12 (2/3): 111–19.

Patrias, D. 1978. *The Sociology of Secret Deviance: The Case of Sexual Sado-masochism.* New York University. (Unpublished manuscript)

Scott, G. G. 1983. *Dominant Women-Submissive Men: An Exploration in Erotic Dominance and Submission.* New York: Praeger Publishers.

Scoville, J. W. 1984. *Sexual Domination Today: Sado-masochism and Domination-submission.* New York: Irvington.

Spengler, A. 1977. "Manifest Sadomasochism of Males: Results of an Empirical Study." *Archives of Sexual Behavior* 6: 441–56.

———. 1979. *Sadomasochisten und ihre subkulturen.* Frankfurt, West Germany: Campus Verlag.

Stekel, W. 1965. *Sadism and Masochism.* New York: Grove Press. (Original work published in 1929)

Weinberg, M. S., C. J. Williams, and C. Moser. 1984. "The Social Constituents of Sadomasochism." *Social Problems* 31: 379–89.

Weinberg, T. S. 1978. "Sadism and Masochism: Sociological Perspectives." *The Bulletin of the American Academy of Psychiatry and the Law* 6: 284–95.

———. 1987. "Sadomasochism in the United States: A Review of Recent Sociological Literature." *Journal of Sex Research* 23: 50–69.

Weinberg, T.S., and G. Falk. 1980. "The Social Organization of Sadism and Masochism." *Deviant Behavior: An Interdisciplinary Journal* 1: 379–93.

Weinberg, T. S., and G. W. L. Kamel. 1983. "S&M: An Introduction to the Study of Sadomasochism," in *S&M: Studies in Sadomasochism,* ed. T. Weinberg & G. W. L. Kamel, pp. 17–24. Amherst, N.Y.: Prometheus Books.

Contributors

NORMAN BRESLOW received his B.F.A. in photography from the Art Center College of Design (Los Angeles), and a B.A. and M.A. in psychology from California State University in Los Angeles. He has written several articles on sadomasochism. He is the author of *Basic Digital Photography* (Focal Press).

JOEL I. BRODSKY taught at the University of Nebraska-Lincoln, where he received his Ph.D. in sociology in 1989. He was interested in the sociology of health and illness, the sociology of lesbians and gay men, social organization, and social inequality. Dr. Brodsky's scholarly work included research on the relationship between gay men and their physicians, AIDS/HIV as a social problem, gay men's health care, and the concept of community among gay men and lesbians. Dr. Brodsky died in April 1994.

PAT CALIFIA is a sex educator and lesbian journalist. She is the author of *Sapphistry: The Book of Lesbian Sexuality* (Naiad Press) and has published extensively in the feminist and gay press.

HAVELOCK ELLIS (1859–1939) was an English physician whose multi-volume work, *Studies in the Psychology of Sex*, revised numerous times over his lifetime, revolutionized the ways in which human sexuality was viewed. Ellis was interested in a wide range of sexuality, not merely in "criminal" or "abnormal" sex. Through the use of case histories, personal experiences, and the observations and reports of anthropologists, physicians, and others, he demonstrated that sexuality could be studied in the same way as other sorts of social behavior. He is recognized as an originator of the scientific study of sex.

LINDA EVANS received her Ph.D. in human sexuality from the University of California, Irvine. She was in the Department of Health and Safety at California State University, Los Angeles.

SIGMUND FREUD (1856–1939), the father of psychoanalysis, has undoubtedly had the greatest impact on our modern attitudes toward human sexuality. Although he did not write specifically about sex as did his contemporary, Havelock Ellis, nevertheless a concern with the importance of sexuality for other areas of human behavior is interwoven throughout his theories of human development.

PAUL H. GEBHARD is an anthropologist and educator. He served as the executive director of the Institute for Sex Research at Indiana University from 1956 to 1983. A colleague of the late Alfred Kinsey, he is the author (with Kinsey) of *Sexual Behavior in the Human Female* (1953); senior author of *Pregnancy, Birth and Abortion* (1958); *Sex Offenders* (1956); and *Kinsey Data: Marginal Tabulations* (1979).

RICK HOULBERG is a professor of broadcast and electronics arts at San Francisco State University. He received his doctorate in mass communication from Ohio State University. Professor Houlberg's research interests include alternative sexual expressions, the history of broadcasting, broadcasting news, and gender representation in broadcasting.

JULIETTE is the pseudonym of a former professional dominatrix and madam who wishes to remain anonymous.

G. W. LEVI KAMEL received a master's degree in sociology from Arizona State University, where he also taught. He earned his doctorate from the University of California, San Diego in 1983. An author of scholarly articles on human sexuality, Dr. Kamel also wrote *Downtown Street Hustlers*. He was the first AIDS Education Services Director for California and also served as a consultant for the California Hemophilia Council. He died from complications of AIDS in 1989.

RICHARD VON KRAFFT-EBING (1840–1902) was a German physician trained as both a neurologist and a psychiatrist. Widely acclaimed in his day, Krafft-Ebing was the author of *Psychopathia Sexualis*, a work that focused upon deviant sexuality. Many of our modern attitudes toward criminality and sexuality may be directly traced to his writings.

JILL LANGLEY received her B.A. in psychology and M.A. in anthropology from California State University, Los Angeles. She also received a M.A. in psychology from UCLA and studied psycholinguistics in the cognitive psychology department.

EUGENE LEVITT, Ph.D., was a professor of clinical psychology in the School of Medicine, Indiana University, Indianapolis. He is deceased.

MARTHA S. MAGILL has done extensive research in the S&M communities in the Northeast. She received her master's degree in cultural anthropology from the University at Buffalo, SUNY, where she is writing her dissertation.

CHARLES MOSER, Ph.D., M.D., is a professor of sexology at the Institute for Advanced Study of Human Sexuality and maintains a private practice specializing in Internal Medicine and Sexual

Medicine in San Francisco. He received his undergraduate education at SUNY at Stony Brook, and an M.S.W. from the University of Washington, a Ph.D. from the Institute for Advanced Study of Human Sexuality, and an M.D. from Hahnemann University. He is board certified in both internal medicine and sexology. S/M continues to be a major focus of his research.

JAMES MYERS was a professor of anthropology at California State University, Chico. He received his Ph.D. from the University of California, Berkeley. His major area of interest is magic, witchcraft, and religion, and he is coauthor (with A. Lehman) of *Magic, Witchcraft, and Religion: An Anthropological Approach to the Supernatural.*

THOMAS S. WEINBERG is a professor of sociology at Buffalo State College. He received his Ph.D. from the University of Connecticut. Dr. Weinberg is the author of numerous professional articles on human sexuality in various scholarly journals. He is the author of *Gay Men, Gay Selves: The Social Construction of Homosexual Identities* (Irvington Publishers) and, most recently, *Gay Men, Drinking, and Alcoholism* (Southern Illinois University Press).

Index